# Lose Weight

# and Keep it Off!

# Lose Weight

# and Keep it Off!

*A Clinical Evidence Based Approach
for Successful Weight Management*

**Matthew Rensberry, M.D., M.B.A.**

ISBN: 978-1-7334356-1-1

# DEDICATION

*To all my patients who have struggled with weight.*

*Thank you for sharing your journey with me, your trust, and your friendship.*

M. R.

# Table of Contents

Preface                                                          ix
1. Introduction                                                   1
   Epidemiology                                                   2
   What Healthy Looks Like                                        3
   Clinically Meaningful Weight Loss                              4
2. Risk Evaluation                                                5
   Comorbidities                                                  6
   Physical Evaluation                                            9
   Laboratory Evaluation                                         10
   Metabolic Syndrome                                            12
3. Establish Your Goals                                          13
   Your Functional Long Term Goal                                13
   Your Short Term (3 months) Objective Goal                     14
   Goal Check-in                                                 15
4. Food Intake                                                   17
   Caloric Restriction                                           18
   Basic Dietary Guidance                                        21
5. Sleep                                                         49
   General Behavioral Strategies to Improve Sleep                52
   Sleep Restriction Therapy                                     54
   Pharmacological Sleep Aids                                    56
   Some Specific Sleep Conditions                                59
6. Stress                                                        65
   Stress Management                                             67
7. Social Aspects of Weight Management                           77
8. Physical Activity                                             79

9.  Medications and Weight Management 85
    Management of Comorbidities 86
    Medications for Weight Loss 98
    Supplements and Over-the-Counter Options for Weight
    Loss 106
10. Bariatric Surgery 113
    Pre-Surgery 114
    Surgical Procedures 115
    Post-op 119
    Body Contouring Surgery 125
11. Final Thoughts 127
12. Appendices 131
    Appendix 1: Weight-Related Calculations 133
    Appendix 2: Smartphone Applications 135
    Appendix 3: Low Glycemic Index Food Reference 139
    Appendix 4: FODMAP Food Reference 153
13. Index 162
About the Author 166
Footnotes 167

# Preface

Excess weight is a disease process similar to how high blood pressure is a disease process. When a person has high blood pressure, they are not treated until their pressure is at goal and then treatment is withdrawn. No, the disease continues to be managed. This same treatment thought process is true with weight as well.

The purpose of this book is multi-factorial. First, it provides a resource for the layperson to understand how extra weight relates to and contributes to disease. Second, this book builds upon that physiologic understanding to provide a strategy for weight loss, improved overall health, and increased functional capacity. Lastly, this book describes insights for weight maintenance after weight loss to prevent weight regain.

In this book, I approach weight management from a lifestyle, whole-person perspective. Achieving and maintaining a healthy weight is a difficult and personal journey that necessitates energy, effort, support, good habits, and persistence. It leads to a more productive and longer life, filled with opportunities. While not easy, it is a worthwhile endeavor.

This book describes the strategy I employ, as I work with my patients, for them to lose weight and maintain their weight loss. While any change can create an effect, no change is, by itself, the only change required. Here I review weight loss strategies and plans that I have successfully employed in clinical practice. The book proceeds in a prioritized order. Within each section, I attempt to provide some of the "why" behind the interventions for weight loss and weight loss maintenance.

This book is a work for empowering others and increasing personal freedom. Living a long active life with the option to enjoy activities without physical restrictions is a life of freedom. This process and journey must be viewed as a lifestyle change, not simply a temporary life adjustment. As you read through this book, consider how it might pertain to your daily life. If you think a change is warranted and you will maintain it long term, do it!

As you read this book, I encourage you to make it personal. Highlight and create a list of changes you can make over time in your own life. Over time, you will be able to start making adjustments which will help you lose weight and help you keep the weight off. We are at the starting line. Your life journey is the fun part

*Matthew Rensberry, MD, MBA*
*Orlando, Florida*

# 1. Introduction

*"If we could give every individual the right
amount of nourishment and exercise, not too
little and not too much, we would have found
the safest way to health."*

*~Hippocrates~*

In the United States, we carry extra weight in the
form of excess fat as a population. This problem began
gradually but has accelerated recently affecting the health
and fitness of a large portion of Americans.

Obesity, defined as a body mass index (BMI) over 30
$Kg/m^2$ does not measure fat directly. Body fat is known to
reflect variably in regards to BMI in different circumstances such as sex, age, race, and Hispanic origin.[1] Not
only does BMI vary within these groups, the morbidity
and mortality associated with these BMI cut points does
as well.

Extra weight contributes to an acceleration of a person's health deterioration as they age. Obesity is associated with conditions such as high blood pressure, cholesterol, blood sugar, liver dysfunction, gall stones, osteoarthritis, depression, various cancers, and more. People find mobility increasingly difficult, exercise tolerance

1

decreased, social discrimination due to weight bias, and potential public embarrassment from everyday situations such as difficulty sitting between armrests.

It can also be expensive to have obesity. The impact of obesity on the healthcare system as a whole is estimated to be quite costly. One study estimated the cost to the United States because of obesity at $147 billion dollars in 2008. At the individual level, the estimated costs for an individual with obesity, compared to someone without extra weight, is an additional $1,429 per year (in 2006)! The increased expense of prescription medications was close to $600 per year for those with obesity compared to normal weight.[2] Achieving and maintaining a healthy weight saves money.

## *1.1. Epidemiology*

Over 36% of all Americans met the criteria for obesity in 2006 with women higher at 39%.[1] Obesity affects all genders, ethnicities, and age groups but disproportionately affects nonhispanic blacks and Hispanic populations.[1] Over the past 30 years, Americans, in general, have been growing heavier. The most likely cause is multifactorial, a collection of many influences in our collective lives and lifestyles. The adjustments we identify in this book will help us reverse many of these causal factors.

Young people have also been affected. In 2014, one-fifth of all teenagers met criteria for obesity.[1] Those who begin life with extra weight in their youth are much more likely to struggle with weight the rest of their life. If 20% of our teenagers currently have obesity, as a community, we will likely continue to have rates over 20% as these teenagers age into adulthood.

Obesity rates are highest in the traditional south portion of the country. Rates are consistent across income and educational levels for men. (In women rates go down with increased income and education level.) The majority of men and women with obesity are above the poverty level.[3] Across all groups, the prevalence of obesity has risen over the past 20 years.

## 1.2. What Healthy Looks Like

What is healthy and what does it look like? We have recognized objective definitions for normal weight, but these definitions do not translate well for individuals in their everyday life. Normal weight is defined as having a BMI between 18.5 $Kg/m^2$ and 24.9 $Kg/m^2$. More importantly, being at a normal BMI does not equate to health. Many normal weight people live unhealthy lifestyles.

Functional abilities and an overall decrease in disease state should really be our definition of health. This means not being restricted from activities you want to do or would like to do because of your health. If you enjoy kayaking, the healthy you not only can go kayaking but is not restricted within the activity. The healthy (kayaking) you does not tire out early, is not restricted in movement, nor lacks the flexibility required to powerfully paddle. If you enjoy running and a friend informs you of a local 5K foot race, a healthy you can go run it on short notice. The healthy you can play sports with your kids and live long enough to see them and your grandchildren grow.

The healthy you needs fewer or no medications. Every medicine has adverse effects, and the fewer required, the less harm they can potentially do to you. As people lose the extra weight they carry, they often require less medicine for diabetes, high blood pressure, cholesterol, pain, and other weight-related conditions.

3

## 1.3. Clinically Meaningful Weight Loss

The good news is just a small reduction in weight can be clinically meaningful. Clinically meaningful means it will have positive effects on comorbidities such as those described.

Clinically meaningful weight loss is losing as little as 5% to 10% of a person's current weight. Losing this amount of body weight improves diabetes mellitus leading to less need for insulin. There is a reduction in cardiovascular disease. Blood pressure improves by as much as 10 mmHg with clinically meaningful weight loss. A loss of just 4 Kg (8.8 lbs) reduces systolic blood pressure by 4.5 mmHg and diastolic blood pressure 3.2 mmHg. Cholesterol improves with decreases is low-density lipoprotein (LDL) and triglyceride levels and a beneficial increase in high-density lipoprotein (HDL) levels. Obstructive sleep apnea can improve up to 50% with a 10% weight loss.[4]

This is an attainable goal and the new beginning of a healthier version of you. This amount of weight loss will assist you to require less medication to control disease, live longer, become more active, and create opportunities for you as you gain functional capacity.

# 2. Risk Evaluation

*"You don't have to be perfect in order to be successful."*

*~Anonymous~*


The first step to address weight is performing a health risk assessment. This identifies modifiable medical concerns where, by addressing these concerns, you might expect improvements. The risk assessment identifies disease processes which you might manage in a different way, and find other reasons why you might find it so difficult to lose weight or keep the weight off. This insight is motivating and helps you focus on the areas where you can affect your personal success.

Many risk factors exist that predispose people to struggle with weight. Some risk factors for obesity have always been out of your control. Genetics have been shown to have a strong influence. A child's weight is associated with parental weight status and BMI, living space, parental educational levels, and parental age.[5]

Intrauterine life affects a person's long term struggle with weight. If a person's mother gained too much weight during her pregnancy, began the pregnancy at a heavier weight, smoked during pregnancy, or developed gestational diabetes, the child is at an increased risk to struggle with weight during their lifetime.

Whether a person was breastfed or not has an effect on their lifelong struggle with weight. Breastfed babies have lower rates of struggling with extra weight, with each month of breastfeeding decreasing their risk by 4%.[6]

Meeting criteria for obesity as an adolescent increases the risk for continued difficulties into adulthood. Poor sleep increases the risk of experiencing a weight struggle, as does increased stress.

These non-modifiable risk factors provide insight into why we struggle with weight. We will concentrate on what we can affect, those aspects where we can make a difference to improve our chances for success in weight loss and then the prevention of weight regain.

## 2.1. Comorbidities

Given the many relationships extra weight shares with so many diseases and disability states, it is important to identify comorbidities to aid optimization of medical management. Carrying extra weight is associated with several diseases and disabilities. Some are related to metabolic changes that occur due to hormonal changes caused by the extra fat cells. Others are related to the physical extra weight from the fat mass itself.

The mass itself, the effects of physically carrying around extra weight, has many potential ramifications.

Carrying around extra weight limits a person's ability to move, restricts their range of motion, and decreases exercise tolerance. It is easier to tire out, and so people find it difficult to walk as far or take the stairs.

Extra weight from the fat mass results in difficulty breathing, gastroesophageal reflux, increased rates of musculoskeletal injuries such as meniscus tears, sprained ankles, and back pain.

The mass can lead to obstructive sleep apnea (OSA) due to the extra weight restricting one's airway. OSA contributes to poor sleep, high blood pressure, and headaches. The extra mass also can lead to abnormal pulmonary function and hypoventilation syndrome as people are unable to fully expand their chest.

In addition to the extra weight evident in the visible areas of our bodies, we also accumulate fat tissue around our organs and within the liver. Non-alcoholic fatty liver disease leads to liver dysfunction due to fat mass accumulation within the liver itself. Over time, this can result in liver cirrhosis.

The mass of extra abdominal weight can cause and worsen acid reflux by increasing the intra-abdominal pressure. Carrying around the extra weight wears on joints, especially knees and back and can develop into osteoarthritis.

The fat cell, called an adipose cell, functions as an endocrine organ itself. Adipose cells produce hormones which affect other body systems. Many hormones from other organs within the body are derived from the same cholesterol molecules stored in adipose cells. As more adipose tissue accumulates within a person's body, higher levels of these hormones are found in circulation. This leads to other physiologic dysfunctions. For instance, the increased estrogen circulating in the body in people with extra weight results in abnormal or absent menstrual cycles, infertility, or body hair changes in women. Higher estrogen levels can result in gynecomastia or low testosterone in men.

Metabolic dysfunction occurs throughout all areas of the body from that involving the small blood vessels (leading to strokes, heart disease, cataracts, erectile dysfunction) to glucose metabolism dysfunction with insulin resistance (diabetes type 2). Other dysfunctions associated with extra weight include gout, gall bladder disease, and psoriasis.[7]

Dysfunction from extra weight also increases cardiovascular diseases such as high blood pressure and high cholesterol. Some disease states both cause and are associated with obesity such as hypothyroidism or polycystic ovarian syndrome (PCOS).

Many cancers are associated with increased weight. Some can be attributed to increased hormone levels, like endometrial, breast, pancreatic, and prostatic cancers. Other cancers associated with extra weight, like colon and esophagus cancers, are potentially dietary related.

Disabilities experienced by those with extra weight include depression and anxiety. People who meet the definitions of overweight and obesity face significant discrimination for that weight.

Genetics plays a role in extra weight as well. Obesity can be inherited and passed on to future generations. Many genetic diseases also are strongly associated with extra weight, such as Prader Willi Syndrome.[7]

You might be diagnosed with one or more of these associated conditions. Improving your weight will help. It can decrease your medication burden as with weight loss, you might require less medicine to control your comorbidities, possibly even discontinue some! It can help maintain function and decrease long term risks from these diseases.

Improving weight management by losing 5% to 10% of body weight is known to be clinically meaningful. This small amount will positively affect your comorbidities, such as their high blood pressure or blood sugar control.

## 2.2. Physical Evaluation

To accurately diagnose your comorbidities and perform a risk assessment, expect your doctor to perform a physical examination. They will look for signs associated with these comorbidities. Things such as skin changes consistent with diabetes (skin tags or darkening of the skin behind the neck called acanthosis nigrans). Other signs they will look for are white skin areas around the eyes that can indicate high cholesterol, frequent urinary tract or vaginal infections, fungal skin infections, neck masses, swollen lymph node, an enlarged liver, small testicles, and more.

Your vital signs provide a good indicator of how your body is managing at the moment. Hypertension manifests with high blood pressure. An increased rate of shallow breathing could indicate restrictive pulmonary function due to extra weight.

Your doctor will want to know your weight and height to calculate your body mass index (BMI). The BMI is a risk stratification tool based on weight and height. People fall into underweight ($<18.5$ Kg/m$^2$), normal weight (18.5-25 Kg/m$^2$), overweight (25-30 Kg/m$^2$), and obesity ($>30$ Kg/m$^2$) categories.[8]

Your waist circumference is another important measurement. This measures your central adiposity, the weight you carry around your mid-section. Reducing your waist circumference is more important than the amount of weight lost over time. It is fat cells in this area which indicate a higher health risk. The waist circumference is performed by measuring the circumference of a person's abdomen on their skin at the level of the umbilicus. The tape should be not too tight and straight across the back. The measurement is taken right after exhaling. A higher waist circumference indicates higher health risks. Cutoffs for higher risk in men is over 40 in, and in women over 35 in.[8]

In the physical exam, it will be important for your doctor to note the distribution type of fat, whether central (often referred to as apple shape) or in hips (often referred to as pear shape). They will look for physical findings that might indicate a disease process such as a fat pad on the back of the neck, purple striae on the abdomen, and widened (moon) face as seen in excess steroid exposure. Other physical findings include any heart rate arrhythmia's, heart murmurs, wheezing in the lungs, overall musculature, skin changes, acne, excessive hair growth, swelling, ulcers, and varicosities.

After a thorough physical exam, a laboratory examination will help complete the assessment.

## 2.3. Laboratory Evaluation

An important and necessary step to identify comorbidities related to extra weight is to obtain laboratory tests. Specific laboratory tests of interest are:

- Fasting blood glucose (FBS)
- Hemoglobin A1c (HbA1c)
- Complete Blood Count (CBC)
- Kidney Function Tests (BUN/Cr)
- Liver Function Tests (LFTs)
- Lipid Profile (Cholesterol)
- Thyroid Stimulating Hormone (TSH)
- Vitamin B12 level (B12)
- Vitamin D level (25-OH)

- Total Testosterone for men (Test)

Fasting blood glucose and HbA1c identify pre-diabetes or diabetes. Pre-diabetes is defined as a FBS over 100 mg/dl or an HbA1c between 5.7% and 6.4%. Diabetes results in higher cutoff points.

The CBC demonstrates any potential anemia. The HbA1c result might need to be taken in context depending on this result as anemia can influence the validity of the HbA1c results.

The kidney function test results will help with medication management. Some medications require renal dosing or should be avoided in those with kidney damage.

Elevated LFTs can indicate, among other disease processes, fatty liver disease (NASH). This is a precursor to fibrosis in the liver which can lead to cancer. The treatment for this condition is weight loss!

People with extra weight are often deficient in vitamin B12 and/or vitamin D. A person with obesity and a B12 level less than 400 pg/ml could benefit from supplementation. Vitamin D, a fat-soluble vitamin, is often low in those with extra weight. If their vitamin D level is less than 30 ng/ml, they should consider supplementation.

Because high insulin levels lead to more weight gain, some providers will obtain an insulin level with the first evaluation. Labs or imaging might be ordered should the physical exam demonstrated a potential reason for inquiry, such as evaluating possible polycystic ovarian disease.

Other laboratory tests can be performed for further evaluation. If needed, these are performed as a secondary set after a positive result from one of those already discussed.

## 2.4. Metabolic Syndrome

Metabolic syndrome is a collection of findings that together indicate an increased health risk. A diagnosis of metabolic syndrome requires three or more of the following:

- Fasting blood glucose above 100 mg/dl
- Blood pressure above 130/85 mm/Hg (or prescribed a hypertension medication)
- Triglycerides above 150 mg/dl
- HDL below 40 mg/dl in men or less than 50 mg/dl in women
- Waist circumference over 102 cm (40 in) in men or 88 cm (35 in) in women

If you meet the criteria for metabolic syndrome, use this diagnosis as motivation for weight loss and loss maintenance. Weight loss will help you mitigate some of the increased health risks metabolic syndrome adds.

# 3. Establish Your Goals

*"People with clear, written goals, accomplish far more in a shorter period of time than people without them could ever imagine."*

*~Brian Tracy~*

The first step towards successful weight management is setting appropriate goals. One tool for successfully achieving goals is to use SMART goals. SMART goals stand for those that are Specific, Measurable, Attainable, Realistic, and Time-bound. Write down each of your goals in this manner. The act of writing your goals down will improve your success. You will need to revisit your goals regularly to check in with yourself and review how your progress is going.

## 3.1. Your Functional Long Term Goal

With weight loss, people improve on their success when they choose long term functional goals over goals of appearance or weight. Avoid choosing a personal goal such as a particular size of clothing or how many pounds you want to lose, and instead, think about what you would like to be capable of doing that your current weight holds you back from fully enjoying. Functional goals can range from being able to complete a 5k foot race, being able to ride a bicycle with your children, or sitting comfortably in an airline seat. Other examples of functional goals could be having the ability to walk a set number of blocks without knee or back pain, garden in your backyard, or not be short of breath when taking a flight of stairs.

Use this goal for motivation. Keep your sights set on it. Over time, you will inch closer and closer to this goal until someday when you reach it. As you progress, new habits will form and you will generate new functional goals. Maintain a list of these. All of these activities will help you maintain the weight loss you achieve during your weight journey.

Make sure to write each goal as a SMART goal. Here is an example of a SMART, long term functional goal for weight loss:

- "I want to be able to walk 4 blocks without getting winded by winter (Specific, Measured, Attainable, Realistic, and Time-bound)."

## 3.2. Your Short Term (3 months)

### Objective Goal

This second goal is a very important goal that will help stay on track with your long term functional goal. The timeframe for this goal is three months. Think of this goal as one step along your journey. Achieving this goal will be motivating. It will help you maintain forward momentum. It will also be an early warning indicator of any struggles or difficulties.

I recommend your first short term goal being your clinically meaningful weight loss amount. Remember a 5% to 10% reduction in weight is clinically meaningful and will make positive improvements on several weight-related medical conditions such as high blood pressure, cholesterol, or blood sugar. Choose a specific amount of weight loss from within that range. You can use the calculator at matthew.rensberry.com to do the math for you.[9]

This amount of weight loss is completely possible. Take the time to write it down now, as in this example:

- I plan to lose 15 lbs over the next 3 months. (A SMART goal)

## 3.3. Goal Check-in

It is important to review the status of your goals regularly. Schedule a formal time for goal review with yourself every month. It is helpful to schedule this in a calendar, take the time to be by yourself free from distractions, and to write down your thoughts. Be honest with yourself during these moments.

Here are some example ideas to jot down:

- How are you doing in regards to your functional long term goal?
- Are you able to walk farther without pain?
- Are you working on climbing stairs when you can?
- Do you get hungry between meals?
- How are you progressing with your short term goal?
- Have you been struggling with a particular intervention?

Decision points line your weight management journey. At times, you will make decisions to continue the current path (when things are progressing according to your overall plan). There will be other times when progress will stall.

At some point, as people lose weight, their weight loss will plateau off. When this happens, you will need to decide whether you have met your goal, what the next lifestyle adjustment or modification to adopt should be, or whether you slipped in your weight management plan in some way and what you need to refocus on. Checking in with yourself regularly will help you stay the course and bring success!

# 4. Food Intake

*"Don't eat anything your great-great grandmother wouldn't recognize as food."*

*~Michael Pollan~*

A calorie is defined as the amount of heat needed to raise a kilogram of water one degree Celsius (4.19 joules). The energy-producing value of food, when oxidized within the body, is expressed in calories.

For many years, weight management was often condensed to a formula of calories in minus calories out. If this equation resulted in a positive value, the person gained weight. If it resulted in a negative value, they lost weight.

This concept has frustrated many who have struggled to lose weight. If it were fully accurate, then losing weight is simply a matter of self-control (restricting calories in) and motivation (exercising to maximize calories out).

An expanding body of evidence demonstrates this is not the case. Much of how much we weigh is affected by things outside of our normal abilities of control. Some examples include hormones and other chemicals in the brain which affect when we feel full, when we are hungry, what we crave, and more.

Importantly, though, not all calories are equal to each other. The caloric energy potential is equally present, but how much your body uses or absorbs can differ between foods. This idea where calories from our diets can be unequal leads to two important points. First, the calorie balance equation, while important, is only a portion of the weight management puzzle. The actual calories you consume, the type of food itself, makes a difference in how your body reacts to the calorie intake.

Let's explore these ideas further.

## 4.1. Caloric Restriction

While no longer the full medical weight management strategy, establishing and maintaining an appropriate caloric restriction is still a critical component to both weight loss and weight loss maintenance.

Evidence supports that those who consume a calorie-restricted diet lose weight, maintain their lower body weight, and live longer.[10] An appropriate calorie restriction is around 500 to 700 calories fewer than needed to maintain your current weight per day.

This number is derived from the idea that a pound of fat is 3,500 calories. Consuming 500 fewer calories a day would lead to a deficit of 3,500 calories over a week. Were your body to use fat cells for those additional 3,500 calories needed to maintain your weight instead of by food intake, you would lose weight.

Since we know not all calories are equal, this is at best only a poor estimate. Still, this estimate is a medically safe one and one which will lead to your long term success in weight loss and maintenance and not lower your metabolism.

It is important to not have too great a calorie deficit. Consuming too few calories can lead to muscle atrophy as your body will use muscle for fuel instead of fat cells. It will slow your metabolism, leading to increased difficulties later with further weight loss, and facilitate weight regain after weight loss. For those reasons, stick to a 500 to 700 calorie deficit unless actively managed by your physician.

Living daily with a caloric restriction has been shown to help people live longer. To do this well, you will need to commit to tracking your calories daily. When a person tracks their food intake, they are mindful of what they consume and automatically take smaller portions. They also avoid some temptations they otherwise might fall for.

You also need to figure out what your daily calorie goal should be. This goal is the number of calories you are trying to eat, not an amount you do not want to go over. Some days you will go over it a little, and other days not, but if things work out well, your daily calorie intake average at the end of the week will be near this number. For most men, this number will be around 1,600 cal/day and women 1,300 cal/day. If you want to use a calculator to figure out this number, you can one online at htttps://matthew.rensberry.com.[9] The calculations can also be found in Appendix 1.

There are a couple of strategies people use to restrict calories. One strategy is to count calories throughout the day as you consume them. This running total continues to provide feedback to let you know how many calories you have left to eat in the day. This can help you plan your next meals and snacks. It can also help give insight into how your body reacts to calories, whether you have cravings at night, or get hungry mid-afternoon, or if you have been eating many more snacks than you thought. With this strategy, it is helpful to add up the estimated calories of your meal before eating it. Doing this helps prevent overeating.

You can add to this strategy by adjusting portion sizes. Adjusting portions allows you to continue to have variety in your diet while consuming fewer calories. Most people do not recognize the serving sizes of their foods. A good habit to develop is reviewing food labels and noting the serving size at the top of the nutrition facts. Over time, as people track their calories and recognize what reported serving sizes are for each food type, they often adjust their portions as well.

A different strategy for calorie restriction, utilizing less tracking, is to remove a disposable calorie item from your diet. After tracking calorie intake for two to three weeks, you can review what you consume to find patterns in consumption. You might find you repeatedly consume certain caloric items you could forgo and live without. For instance, you might use less creamer (40 cal/creamer) or sugar (15 cal/tsp) in your daily coffee. You could stop all soda (140 cal/12 oz) consumption.

Try to not drink calories and instead enjoy your calories in solid foods. Drink fluids like black coffee, unsweetened tea, water, or unsweetened flavored carbonated water. This is an individualized decision and will not be successful for all people. One patient of mine lost 30 pounds simply by decreasing the amount of coffee she drank in a day instead of decreasing the amount of creamer and sugar in each coffee. She simply drank less of the same excessively sweet and creamy coffee.

To track your calorie intake, find a system that works for you. One you can use for the long term. Many smartphone applications exist to help in this regard (See Appendix 2). Tracking calories on paper also works fine. At first, tracking seems like a chore, but with practice, like all things, it gets easier and more intuitive.

By this point, you have determined your long term functional goals, your short term (3 months) objective goal, a daily caloric goal, and a strategy to meet that daily calorie goal. Let's discuss dietary choices further.

## 4.2. Basic Dietary Guidance

In this section, we will discuss some general dietary guidance along with the reasoning behind the recommendations. This section is important because diet is quite influential in affecting weight loss. Of all weight affecting modalities, it is the most influential for change.

## 4.2.1. Recommendation: Consume less processed foods

We know that weight management is much more than the simple equation of calories in minus calories out to lose (or gain) weight. Put another way, not all calories are the same. Our bodies react to calories from different foods differently.

One calorie from an apple is different than a calorie from a glazed doughnut. When we consume the apple calorie, our bodies absorb the sugar in a gradual and controlled manner, whereas with a doughnut, our blood glucose spikes as our bodies rapidly absorb the sugar. This rate of rise is important as, our bodies use insulin, secreted from our pancreas, to bring the glucose level back down to normal levels.

Insulin is a hormone secreted by the pancreas in response to feeding. Its role is to control the glucose level in the bloodstream by lowering it. Insulin is secreted when your body tastes food and the flavor of sweetness. One way insulin brings down the bloodstream glucose level is it helps facilitate glucose entering the cells of muscles and other tissues who use them for energy. These tissues, such as muscles, then preferentially use this glucose and glycogen for energy, over the body's stored fat energy.

Insulin also lowers glucose in the bloodstream by converting glucose in the liver to glycogen (another energy storage molecule). Then, when the liver is saturated with glycogen, additional glucose is shunted to make fatty acids, which the fat cells use to make triglycerides. (This increase in triglycerides can lead to atherosclerosis development). In this way, insulin brings down the glucose levels in the bloodstream through fat synthesis. It helps turn the glucose into stored fat.

These mechanisms of insulin function demonstrate how insulin has a fat-sparing effect. It encourages the body to both avoid the breakdown of existing fat by pushing glucose into tissues to be used preferentially for energy use first, and then indirectly stimulates the growth of fat cells.

Insulin is one of only two hormones (the other is leptin) that function as long term signals to the brain of adiposity (body fat). This means the level of insulin in the body helps the brain regulate food intake to restore adipose (fat) tissue to a regulated level. As insulin levels rise, neurons in the hypothalamus of the brain are inhibited which deactivate the feeding response. Insulin levels are proportional to the dysfunction of the body fat (adiposopathy).

What allows for the sugar in apples to be absorbed in a more controlled manner within the body is the amount of fiber. Foods with fiber require more energy for digestion compared with foods that lack dietary fiber (such as donuts). The fiber also blunts the sugar spike that would otherwise occur. This blunted spike in glucose results in a similar comparative blunting in the rise of insulin. More fiber-rich foods leads to less immediate (and more importantly cumulative) exposure to insulin and its fat synthesis effects. Fiber also lowers total calorie absorption, meaning a lower percentage of calories are absorbed from the apple due to its inherent fiber content than the doughnut with its lack of fiber content.

Note, this is not added fiber, but the fiber that comes from the food itself. This is important, as adding fiber has been shown to not help people lose weight. Fiber from unprocessed foods, conversely, is associated with weight loss. The effect is different between inherent fiber content and added fiber. The added fiber does not carry the same effect.

The practical application of these ideas suggests we should consume a higher proportion of our meals as unprocessed fruits and vegetables. Concentrating on adding fruits and vegetables to your diet will improve nutritional quality and your glucose homeostasis, especially when they are not processed.

In the processing of foods, much of the fiber (and color) is removed. A lot of its nutritional content is also removed while retaining the sweetness of the food. In the processing, much of the nutritional content is lost with many of the important vitamins and minerals lost in the portions that are processed off. For these reasons, a good rule is to avoid white foods, such as white bread. White bread has lost much of its fiber and nutritional quality compared to brown whole grain bread. The same goes for white rice compared with brown rice.

Another example is to choose sweet potatoes over regular potatoes. They have more fiber and are more nutritious. In general, we eat too many potatoes. They are the most consumed vegetable in the US, and often in calorie-dense, highly processed forms such as french fries or potato chips.

Preparing and cooking meals at home can help lower your processed food intake. When you cook your own meals, you have full control over what goes into it. Cooking at home carries other benefits as well. Home-cooked meals can be a more economical option and provide positive family experiences.

# 4.2.2. Recommendation: Minimize added sugars

We, as a culture, have developed a sugar addiction. Almost every food has been sweetened in some way. As far as nutrition goes, your body does not need any carbohydrates from added sugars. Thus, all added sugars are unnecessary for a healthy body. This is why most food guidance recommends using added sugars sparingly, if at all.

As we discussed earlier, insulin works to lower glucose (sugar) in the bloodstream by pushing it into cells for energy use (like muscle cells) and through fat accumulation within fat cells. Adding sugars to your diet will increase your cumulative insulin levels.

The average added sugar intake for Americans is 88 grams (22 teaspoons) of sugar a day.[11] This is an unnecessary and additional 350 calories a day for most Americans! The majority of this added sugar comes from processed foods such as cereals and sugar-sweetened beverages.

For guidance, the American Heart Association (AHA) recommends that women do not consume more than 100 calories (24 grams) a day from added sugars and men no more than 150 calories (36 grams) a day.[12]

Our added sugars come from candy, cakes, cookies, pies and cobblers, sweet rolls, pastries, donuts, dairy desserts like ice cream, and sugar-sweetened beverages. Half of our added sugars come from sugar-sweetened beverages.[13]

Your body metabolizes all sugars the same way, whether they come from white sugar, brown sugar, cane sugar, or high fructose corn syrup. It is important to develop the habit of reading food labels to spot these added sugars. Knowing that every gram of sugar is four calories makes calculating the calories from added sugars simple as the standard food labels state how many grams of sugar are included.

Sugar-sweetened beverages are drinks such as regular soft drinks, energy drinks, sports drinks, and fruit drinks (including juices). Our bodies register liquid calories from carbohydrates (sugars) differently than solid foods. Liquid calories are less filling. You remain feeling hungry despite consuming calories in the drink.[14] For adults, each additional daily 12 ounce serving of fruit juice has an associated 24% higher all-cause mortality risk.[15]

Many regular sodas or fruit drinks are 150 to 160 calories. This is about 40 grams of added sugar (or close to 10 teaspoons)! A strategy, if you enjoy soda, is to switch to seltzer, club soda, or sparkling water. This allows for refreshing hydration that still feels like a treat!

There are many names for sugar found on nutrition labels. Some names end in "ose" such as sucrose or fructose. Other added sugars are named anhydrous dextrose, molasses, cane sugar, syrup, honey, nectar, fruit juice concentrate, among others.

Using the calculation of 3,500 calories being equal to a pound of fat, drinking one additional sugar-sweetened beverage with 150 calories a day without any other adjustment in caloric intake will result in a gain of over a pound every month!

It is wise to develop the habit of reviewing nutrition facts labels on foods. It is also good to avoid consuming liquid calories such as those found in sugar-sweetened beverages.

Let's quickly discuss artificial sweeteners. You might think that since artificial sweeteners have no calories, they could sweeten things without creating weight concerns. Unfortunately, artificial sweeteners, such as those found in diet sodas, are associated with weight gain, not weight loss. While there are some theories as to why this happens, the evidence as to why this occurs is quite limited.

One thought is related to the hormonal response in relationship to calories. The body responds to an expected caloric intake when the sweet taste receptors are stimulated. Sweet taste receptors are stimulated by both sugar and artificial sweeteners. With the use of artificial sweeteners over time, the body's response to calories is diminished. It learns not all sweet sensations are calories. When calories are consumed, the body is less responsive and the person does not feel full as soon as they should. In this way, artificial sweeteners trick our bodies into consuming more calories than we should.

Another suggested explanation is that artificial sweeteners change the bacterial composition of the gut. These sweeteners have been demonstrated to kill off beneficial gut bacteria.[16] This gut flora plays a critical role in digestion and absorption of nutrients. The disruption of this gut microbiome might interfere with how sugar is metabolized and even to what extent a person might desire or crave sugar.

A prudent food choice is to avoid all artificial sweeteners. In general, choose sugar over artificial sweeteners, and use less of it. If you want sweetened coffee, use sugar and count those calories as added sugar calories in your

26

tracking. If you want a sweetened soda, drink regular soda and count those calories as added sugar calories in your calorie tracking. Though again, try not to drink calories.

Examples of artificial sweeteners are:

*   aspartame

*   acesulfame-K

*   saccharin

*   sucralose

*   neotame

*   advantame

## 4.2.3. Recommendation: Don't worry too much about a specific diet

When people adopt a diet for weight loss, they will lose weight regardless of diet. Some popular diets concentrate on macro-nutrient composition. This means concentrating on the percentage of fat, carbohydrates, and protein a person consumes. Other diets concentrate on types of food. Some diets concentrate on consuming only food items that result in a particular effect on the body. Others help manage comorbidities.

In this section, consider how your body responds to the foods you consume. What we eat has a direct effect on our body's hormone regulation of weight. Think about how you can adjust your usual food consumption in such a way that you can continue this dietary pattern for the long term (making a lifestyle change).

Use this section as a resource to make purposeful changes with sound reasoning behind them. Write your plan down. Discuss it with your friends and family. These actions will help you commit, gain accountability, and be successful in your weight management.

### Low Carbohydrate Diets (Atkins, Keto, South Beach)

One popular diet category is the low carbohydrate diet. With these diets, people limit their total carbohydrate intake in the hopes their body will burn fat for energy while the person does not feel hungry. There is evidence that those using a low-carbohydrate diet, increase energy expenditure during weight loss maintenance.[17] This indicates that a low carbohydrate diet is a reasonable choice for those who lost weight, to keep it off. It also might benefit those who have diabetes or pre-diabetes, as limiting carbohydrates can benefit those disease processes.

Cholecystokinin (CCK) is a hormone released in the first part of our intestines in response to the consumption of fatty acids (fats and proteins). CCK affects the gastrointestinal system by stimulating the gallbladder and pancreas to release bile and other digestive enzymes. These work to digest fats and proteins. CCK also regulates appetite (energy intake) through receptors in the hypothalamus in the brain, resulting in both a slowing down of the food transit through the gastrointestinal system and earlier sensation of satiety (feeling full).

One popular low-carbohydrate diet, the Keto diet, is a slightly more extreme low carbohydrate diet. This diet severely restricts the total carbohydrates allowed per day often to less than 20g and encourages calories to come from foods with higher fat content. This diet pushes the body into a state of ketosis where its energy is derived from fats rather than sugar. Historically, a ketogenic diet has been used to manage some seizure disorders and has been found to be helpful in Alzheimer's and Parkinson's diseases. Increasing fats in a person's diet will often lead

28

to calorie restriction due to the resulting increased satiety. The digestion of fats also assists with the absorption of some other nutrients.

When consuming a low-carbohydrate diet, you increase the consumption of fats and proteins. These stimulate the release of CCK, helping you to feel full sooner (satiety). CCK also slows down how fast the food progresses through your intestines, helping you feel full longer.

### Low-Fat Diet

Another popular diet is the low-fat diet. In this diet, people limit their total fat intake. This diet was recommended by the US Federal Government initially in a 1977 report titled "Dietary Goals" where it encouraged people to increase consumption of items like fruits, vegetables, whole grains, poultry, and fish while minimizing meats, eggs, and high-fat foods. In the following years, this opinion was given further support by the American Society of Clinical Nutritionists, the American Heart Association (AHA), and the National Cancer Institute. Throughout the 1980s and 1990s, a consensus built among the scientific community promoting low-fat diets.[18]

Fat has nine calories per gram compared with four calories per gram in protein and carbohydrates. People could potentially consume a higher volume of food, consisting of more protein and carbohydrates relatively while taking in a similar amount of calories.

The popularity of this diet changed the food industry's processing of food and later the general public's food consumption habits. In the 1990s, the AHA began to label low-fat foods with a "heart-healthy" label. Producers could purchase this label to add a health credibility for their products. These and other actions resulted in increased consumption of fat-free foods where the fats were substituted with highly processed and refined carbohydrates.

Consumption of these highly processed and refined carbohydrates is problematic as it leads to increased inflammatory states. One link between obesity and insulin resistance, such as in diabetes, is low-grade chronic inflammation. This inflammation occurs as early as three weeks of eating refined carbohydrates.[19] Consumption of refined carbohydrates is a risk factor for insulin resistance (diabetes), independent of central adiposity (fat).[20]

Additionally, refined carbohydrates lead to increased portion sizes due to delayed satiety. There is evidence supporting a change in serotonin signaling within the brain in those who eat more refined carbohydrates. These changes in hormone signaling lead to changes in both satiety and hunger signals.[21] This explains why people sometimes struggle to stop eating some feel-good food items such as white bread or potato chips.

Leptin is a hormone made by our white adipose (fat) cells. It signals to the brain the status of our energy storage, or fat, level. At a certain level, it tells the brain there is sufficient energy storage for normal daily activities. As fat cells decrease, as in weight loss, the level of leptin decreases as well. This signals that the body's energy storage is too low. The brain reacts by initiating activities to regain energy storage and to reaccumulate fat.

Some people develop leptin resistance. When this happens, the brain of people with excess fat (and thus high leptin) does not recognize the elevated leptin level. While the person might have obesity, their brain acts as if they still need additional energy storage. At low levels of leptin, food is a rewarding experience. Elevated leptin should indicate to the brain that a person does not need to eat and can feel full. With leptin resistance, this cerebral reward system fails.

Refined carbohydrates lead to insulin spikes and chronic inflammation. These develop insulin resistance, which in turn leads to leptin resistance. Insulin and leptin resistance result in weight gain and obesity. Minimize refined carbohydrates to avoid obesity.

The idea of low-fat foods being the key to good nutrition was extensively promoted. Over time, research has shed new light onto the different types of fats and the danger of substituting refined carbohydrates for fats in food. The scientific community slowly began to embrace other diets, such as the Mediterranean diet, as a heart-healthy diet.[18]

People do lose weight with low-fat diets. Also, heart disease decreased concurrently with the popular adoption of the low-fat diet. It is important to not substitute high-fat foods with low-fat alternative foods that are highly processed or contain refined carbohydrates. Instead, consume foods that are low-fat in their unprocessed state.

### Vegan/Vegetarian/Flexitarian Diets

People choose to follow a vegetarian or vegan diet for many reasons. There are religious, cultural, political, climate, animal concerns, and many other reasons to minimize or avoid eating animal or animal products. Compared to meat-eaters, people who eat vegan or vegetarian diets both live longer (6 to 9 years longer) and have lower rates of obesity.[22,23]

Consuming more vegetables helps you reach satiety sooner. Vegetables have a lower caloric density than many other foods. They take up more space in your stomach while bringing fewer calories along comparably.

Hunger and satiety are modulated through several hormonal mechanisms. Ghrelin, the hunger hormone, is released in the fundus of the stomach in response to an empty stomach. An empty stomach increases the ghrelin in your body, increasing the hunger sensation you feel. There is a surge just before a meal. Ghrelin levels rise with fasting as well. Other situations that increase ghrelin levels are increased stress and sleep deprivation.

As you eat, your stomach stretches with food and ghrelin secretion is inhibited. Ghrelin levels decrease after meals contributing to the sensation of satiety. Satiety is the term describing the feeling of fullness after a meal. For those with obesity, the amount of Ghrelin decrease after a meal is attenuated compared to those without obesity.

Consuming more vegetables allows for you to stretch your stomach, inhibiting ghrelin release, and helps you feel satiated with fewer calories. Vegetable consumption, with its higher fiber content, results in smaller insulin spikes and decreased rates of insulin resistance (diabetes) among vegetarians.[24]

Often, between meals, your ghrelin levels might rise, leading you to desire a snack. Substituting vegetables, like carrots, instead of potato chips, will help you feel full by distending your stomach and decreasing your ghrelin levels. This decreases your feeling of hunger. At the same time, you consume fewer calories (than you would have with chips) with a more nutritious snack. The added fiber in the carrots will help to avoid both glucose and insulin spikes.

### Glycemic Index Diet

For those with diabetes, one dietary strategy is the low glycemic index diet. The glycemic index (GI) is a measure indicating the amount a type of food affects the rise in blood glucose levels. Foods with a lower GI value are digested more slowly and cause a slower, lower total rise in blood glucose and insulin.

When you consume a low GI food diet, the food is more likely to provide energy for you rather than be stored in fat. Low glycemic index foods help decrease your ghrelin levels by stretching your stomach, while not increasing your insulin levels as much as higher GI foods would. There is evidence that a person can lose weight by eating low GI foods instead of high GI foods, even when the calorie intake remains the same.

The GI value of a food can be affected in several ways. For instance, how long a food is cooked (al dente pasta has a lower GI value), or how ripe it is (ripe fruit have higher GI value) can change the GI value. The presence of acids or fats along with the food, like the addition of vinegar or lemon juice, will lower the GI value. The more surface area of a food, like in small refined flour particles and puffed, fluffy bread, the higher the GI value. The level of refinedness or processing of a carbohydrate also affects the GI value.

A low GI diet is beneficial for those with diabetes, with high cholesterol, and even for weight maintenance.[25,26] It is a potentially long term sustainable diet.

To start a low GI diet, you would evaluate what types of foods you typically eat, identify which ones are high GI foods, and find a substitute with a lower GI value. Low GI foods are defined as those with a value of 55 or less, medium GI foods are between 56 and 69, and high GI foods are 70 and above. You can see a sample list of GI values for some select foods in Appendix 3 or online at matthew.rensberry.com.

### FODMAP Diet

Many people experience chronic gastrointestinal symptoms and search for a diet that can help them manage their symptoms and weight. A low FODMAP diet might help. This diet consists of minimizing the consumption of Fermentable Oligosaccharides, Disaccharides, Monosaccharides, and Polyols (FODMAPs). This diet has been shown to improve symptoms for many gastrointestinal diseases such as irritable bowel syndrome (IBS), functional gastrointestinal syndrome (FGS), small intestinal bacterial overgrowth (SIBO), some auto-immune disorders, inflammatory bowel disease (like Crohn's or ulcerative colitis), and others.[27]

The low FODMAP diet is a temporary restrictive elimination diet where after a period of time, some foods are reintroduced into the person's regular diet. To use this diet, for up to eight weeks, you would eat as few FODMAPs as possible. Then, you would introduce one food type at a time to see what triggers symptoms. Once you know what foods cause symptoms, you avoid all those trigger foods.

Addressing these common gastrointestinal complaints can help a person on a weight journey to gain control over their health and daily function. You can find a list of high and low FODMAP foods in Appendix 4 or online at matthew.rensberry.com.

### Very Low-Calorie Diet

Weight loss clinics will sometimes employ a very low-calorie diet (VLCD) where a person temporarily changes from a normal diet to one of shakes, drinks, or bars. While on these diets, people will consume less than 800 calories a day. It is important to only follow a VLCD with the supervision of a physician. It is critical a person maintains a nu-

34

tritional balance when on such a restrictive diet. A VLCD should only be undertaken for a short time frame, such as a few weeks.

VLCDs are best for people with severe obesity who need to lose a significant amount of fat mass. This diet attempts to push the body to obtain all (or most) its energy from the fat cells instead of using glucose from the diet.

People on a VLCD can lose weight very quickly. While on a VLCD, they will need to take supplements and undergo frequent blood tests to evaluate their electrolytes, blood sugar, blood cell counts, micronutrients, as well as blood pressure.

While on a VLCD, people do not take in enough calories to support exercise. With such a substantial caloric restriction, their bodies will be trying to obtain energy from any source, including muscles. To prevent or minimize muscle breakdown for energy, people on a VLCD consume high protein portions. Muscle loss is an adverse effect of using a VLCD.

In the brain, there is an area with a collection of nerves named the arcuate nucleus. Within the arcuate nucleus there are receptors for a protein called Cocaine-and-Amphetamine-regulated-transcript (CART). This protein's levels are affected in response to leptin, CCK, and Neuropeptide Y (NPY) levels. Increased CART levels suppress food intake. Lower activity of CART in depressed animals is associated with increased food consumption and weight gain.[28] This might be a reason why we gain weight when we are depressed.

When people consume too few calories, this food deprivation leads to a reduction in the arcuate nucleus expression of CART. People lose some of the anorexin (weight loss) effects of CART. This is why consuming too few calories can still result in weight gain.

The adverse effects of being on a VLCD include gall-stones, dry mouth, fatigue, constipation, diarrhea, headache, dizziness, muscle cramps, and hair loss. Very importantly, using a VLCD to lose weight slows down a person's metabolism as their bodies try to conserve all the energy they can. This slower metabolism is partly due to the decreased CART expression in the brain.

People can lose a significant amount of weight quickly on VLCDs (3 to 5 lbs per week/44 lbs over 12 weeks), but they often gain the weight back over time. Having a re-sulting slower metabolism makes weight regain easier and further weight loss difficult.

These diets are very difficult to sustain. The VLCD is a diet best reserved for those with severe morbid obesity who must lose weight quickly to qualify for a surgery, for potential fertility treatment, or to help rapidly address a medical condition such as diabetes. These diets are dras-tic and are not a first-line option.

### Other Diets

When browsing a bookstore for dietary advice, there is an enormous amount of diets to choose from with many varied opinions on the matter. As already discussed, there is quite some overlap among these diets for weight loss. Occasionally, there are diets specifically for conditions of-ten associated with extra weight.

Examples of such diets include the Mediterranean and DASH Diet. These diets might work well for those with a family history or who personally have hypertension (high blood pressure), coronary artery disease, or diabetes. Peo-ple lose weight on these diets, especially when they main-tain an appropriate caloric restriction.

The Mediterranean diet is not a diet so much as a way to eat. The diet itself de-emphasizes red meat, sugar and saturated fat while encouraging fruits, vegetables, whole grains, beans, nuts, legumes, olive oil, and other healthy foods. People on this diet might consume fish and seafood a couple of times a week. They eat chicken, eggs, and cheese in moderation. A glass of red wine daily is not discouraged in this diet.

The dietary approaches to stop hypertension (DASH) diet was designed specifically to address hypertension. It emphasizes similar foods such as fruits, veggies, whole grains, lean protein, and low-fat dairy. The DASH diet recommends avoiding or limiting foods high in saturated fats and added sugars. Additionally, the DASH diet limits salt (sodium) intake initially to less than 2,300 mg a day and eventually less than 1,500 mg a day. Most sodium that we consume comes from packaged foods. Check nutrition labels to limit your sodium intake.

Both of these diets are sustainable over the long term. These diets are not difficult to adopt and have many resources available.[29,30,31]

### Diet Summary

This short diet review did not cover all diets, but you can use the information presented to evaluate any diet you might consider adopting. When it comes to weight loss, regardless of food choices, the most important factor common to all successful diets is maintaining a calorie restriction. Body-weight change is primarily dependent on a calorie deficit and not the composition of macro-nutrients. After a year, people lose about the same amount of weight on low-fat diets as low-carbohydrate diets (about 11.6 – 13.2 lbs).[32]

People will lose weight, in the short term, on most diets and we have discussed a few of the many reasons for this effect. A different, but important question, is how to maintain the weight loss over the long term. This answer is individualized. The best dietary choices for each person are the lifestyle changes that can be maintained long term for that person. Short term dietary adjustments, which are not sustainable, will not continue to work for you. Regardless of your choice of diet and dietary adjustments, make each choice purposely as one you expect to sustain for life.

# 4.2.4. Recommendation: When you eat is also important

When a person eats, their body enters a fed state. In this state, the body obtains its energy from the consumed food only. The body takes excess energy, and using insulin, stores it into fat cells around the body. This fed state lasts approximately three hours after eating.

Following the fed state, the body enters a post-absorptive state, also called the early fasting state. This period lasts from the end of the fed state to about 12 to 18 hours after a meal.

While in the fed state, insulin inhibits a hormone called glucagon. This balance adjusts as the body enters the early fasting state where glucagon levels rise while insulin levels drop. Throughout this time in the fasting state, the body obtains energy through several processes.

Glycogen is a molecule of energy storage, created from glucose in consumed food and stored in the liver and skeletal muscle. This process of glycogen storage is a result of insulin during the fed state. Rising glucagon levels work on the liver to break glycogen molecules down into glucose for the body to use as energy. This process is called glycogenolysis.

The glycogen stored in the muscle cells is available to those muscles but not to the body as a whole. The liver stores about 25% of the body's glycogen storage which can be depleted within 24 hours of starvation.

Another energy production process occurring during this post-absorptive timeframe is gluconeogenesis. This entails the production of glucose out of lactate, alanine, glutamine, and glycerol molecules. Glucagon mediates this process which also takes place within the liver.

Between meals, triglycerides stored in fats cells are broken down into fatty acid molecules. These fatty acids are then used by cells around the body to produce energy molecules through a process called beta-oxidization.

Byproducts of beta-oxidation include multiple molecules containing a chemical structure called a ketone. These molecules are collectively called ketone bodies. Ketone bodies are produced by the liver in times of fasting, starvation, prolonged intense exercise, during low carbohydrate diets, and occasionally in Type 1 Diabetes.

Ketones can be used by mitochondria containing cells to produce energy. Unlike fatty acids, they can reach the brain and be used for energy. They are thus a viable substitute for fuel in the brain during periods of fasting, starvation, intense exercise, and other times when glucose levels might be lower than normal. Short periods of fasting can stimulate the use of fat for energy while not stimulating a change in metabolism.

There are several ways to take advantage of how the body uses fats for fuel to help improve the ratio of fat-to-nonfat mass. One strategy is to restrict food consumption on two non-consecutive days of the week completely or to less than 600 calories while eating in the usual manner the other five days. This dietary strategy is often called the 5:2 Diet.

A different strategy is to consume all the daily calories within an eight to ten-hour window and not eat for the other 14 to 16 hours of the day. This diet is commonly called the 16:8 Diet.

Another simple and sustainable way to incorporate intermittent fasting into daily life is to not eat within three hours of going to bed. This, combined with the time spent sleeping, helps to lengthen the daily fasting state.

The timing inherent in these eating strategies provides a fasting period intended to lower the overall cumulative insulin levels while increasing the amount of energy obtained from fat storage.

Intermittent fasting beneficially affects fat cell metabolism through increased insulin sensitivity, lower leptin levels, and raised adiponectin levels. Combined with exercise, intermittent fasting improves the action of insulin resulting in less overall insulin exposure.[33]

## 4.2.5. Recommendation: Shop for groceries around the outer perimeter

We have already discussed the importance of natural fiber in our dietary choices. Generally, this means less processed foods are healthier foods. In most grocery stores, the inner area of the store tends to hold many of the processed foods. The produce and other less processed foods will be around the outer perimeter of the store.

An emerging body of evidence is growing on the importance of a person's microbiome as it relates to weight management. The microbiome is a term used to describe the collection and mix of bacteria within a person's gastrointestinal tract. The microbiome holds some influence over how food is digested and calories are absorbed as food passes through the gut.

The two dominant phylum of bacteria in humans are Firmicutes and Bacteroidetes. The ratio of these two types of bacteria within the human microbiome is thought to contribute to the person's overall weight.

Those with extra weight tend to have more Firmicutes and fewer Bacteroidetes while those with normal weight have a higher ratio of Bacteroidetes compared with Firmicutes.

People with obesity also have lower functional diversity of bacteria due to the abundance of Firmicutes in their microbiome. In animal models, increases in the Firmicutes proportion of the gut microbiome led to an increase in both the sizes of fat droplets digested as well as the total amount.[34] Studies have also demonstrated the number of Firmicutes is inversely proportional to that of Bacteroidetes.[35]

As a person loses weight, there is a change in their microbiome to decrease the proportion of Firmicutes and increase that of Bacteroidetes.[36] This change in bacterial flora can occur rapidly. It is evident in those on a low-fat diet after a 6% weight loss and for those on a low carbohydrate diet after a 2% loss of weight.

Consuming more unprocessed foods shifts this bacterial ratio in a positive direction. Prioritizing and predominantly shopping the perimeter of a store will help with food purchase choices.

Frozen and canned produce can be as nutritious as fresh produce. They can also be convenient and affordable options. Purchase those without sugary syrups or salty sauces by checking labels and choosing those with the lowest amounts of sodium and added sugars.

41

## 4.2.6. Recommendation: Learn portion sizes and work on portion control

Portion sizes have grown along with the American waistline. For instance, both the standard bagel size and the average serving of spaghetti and meatballs have doubled since the 1970s.[37] Learning to recognize what the expected portion size is for a particular food is critical to optimal caloric intake.

Several factors influence portion consumption. In general, we have lost our context of what a normal portion size is. The only way to achieve portion control is to put in the effort to learn what the appropriate portion size is for the food consumed. This requires reading food labels, practice, and time.

Serving size and portion size are similar but different terms. Serving size is noted on nutrition labels to identify the number of calories per amount typically eaten in a setting. Portion size is the amount actually consumed. When trying to control caloric intake, you might eat less or more than the serving size listed to accomplish your goals. The nutritional description of the serving size serves as a guide to help you understand how many calories, carbohydrates, added sugars, sodium, protein, and fats you consume in your portion.

Sometimes this size is described by a number, for instance, a serving size of pretzels might be 20 pretzels. Other times, the size is weight, such as if a portion of pretzels is 30 grams. This suggests a food scale could be a handy tool to keep in the kitchen. Occasionally, the serving size is volume, as in a can of soda might be one can.

As the serving size and portion size can vary depending on food type, who produces the food, and other factors, it is helpful to have some portion size guidelines.

Here is an easy guide to estimate portion sizes. Use this guide when filling your plate and choosing what to eat:

- 1/2 cup (125 ml) = 1/2 closed fist
  - Fresh, frozen or canned fruit
  - Fresh, frozen or canned vegetables
  - Fruit juice
- 1 cup (250 ml) = 1 closed fist
  - Cold cereal (30 g)
  - Leafy vegetables
  - Legumes (175 ml)
  - Milk
  - Pasta
  - Rice
  - Whole fruit
  - Yogurt (175 ml)
- 1/4 cup (60 ml) = 1 level cupped hand
  - Nuts
  - Pretzels
- 2 1/2 ounces (75 g) = the palm of your hand
  - Meat
  - Fish
  - Poultry
- 1 teaspoon (5 ml) = 1 thumb tip
  - Margarine or butter
  - Oil
  - Mayonnaise
- 1 tablespoon (15 ml) = 1 thumb
  - Cheese (2 tbsp, 1 oz, or 30 ml)

- Honey
- Margarine or butter
- Mayonnaise
- Oil
- Peanut butter
- Salad dressing (2 tbsp, 1 oz, or 30 ml)

Portion control requires planning. One strategy that helps with portion control is to prepare meals ahead of time in the correct portion sizes. This can be performed at the beginning of each week, frozen or refrigerated, and make for simple meals.

Another way to control portions is through a portion plate. These are relatively inexpensive tools to help guide how much food of different types to place on your plate for each meal. They have sections labeled and sized for fruits or vegetables, starch or grains, and protein.

Even without a portion plate, you can use plate size to help you and your family psychologically make better portion size choices. For instance, try using larger plates for the salad and smaller plates for the main meal.

Often, people will eat more of a food if it comes from a larger package. For this reason, it can be a good habit to divide up a package into smaller containers to avoid over-consumption. Similarly, avoid eating straight from the package, using an appropriately sized container instead.

People will eat what is more easily available. When eating at home, do not leave the food on the table, have people get up to serve themselves. This will help curb consumption.

If it is out of sight or not in the home, it will not be eaten. Replace a candy dish with a fruit bowl. You can move tempting foods such as cookies or ice cream to high shelves or the back of the freezer. Place better food choices in easier to access locations such as at eye level or on the counter.

Learning what an appropriate serving size is and controlling portion sizes will lead to control over calorie intake. Mindfulness of portion size at each meal will improve your nutritional intake as well.

# 4.2.7. Recommendation: Have a strategy for eating out

One of the biggest temptations for dietary indiscretions occurs when we eat outside the home. It is more economical and more nutritious to eat home-prepared meals. Frequency of eating out is directly correlated with BMI. The more a person eats outside the home, especially at fast-food restaurants, the more calories and fat intake they consume and heavier they are.[38] It is a good idea to limit eating out to less than once a week.

We often find ourselves away from home, short on time, or going out to eat for nice occasions. Successful weight management requires a plan before heading out to eat.

Restaurants, in general, serve larger portions of calorie-dense foods today than ever before. Choosing wisely at a restaurant can be difficult as more nutritious and healthier foods might not be as tempting as those that are less so.

Here are some helpful techniques when eating out:

- When ordering your meal:
  - Look up the menu before you go to the restaurant and have a plan. Develop a plan for locales you commonly frequent.
  - When deciding what to order, choose protein such as fish, chicken, or plant-based foods like

tofu and avoid carbohydrates like pasta, rice, or potatoes.

- You can choose an appetizer as your main meal to help assure your portion size is reasonable.

- If your order comes with a starch, choose one with a lower glycemic index. Alternatively, you can ask to substitute the starch with more vegetables.

- Choose to drink water or unsweetened tea

- When at buffet-style restaurants, as you plate your food, fill half of your plate with vegetables and salad. Split the other half of the plate into 2/3 protein and 1/3 carbohydrates.

- Restaurants will often lure people with more food for less money. Should you recognize they are simply adding more starch such as pasta, french fries, or rice, pass on the deal.

- When eating your meal:

  - People will consume more when they are served larger portions. At the beginning of your meal, request a box for you to take half of your meal home. Place half in the box before eating. You could instead share the meal with someone else.

  - Eat your meal slowly. Consumption speed affects satiety regulation. If you are accustomed to eating fast, slowing down can be difficult. Try placing your silverware down between bites. Being mindful of the tastes, and thoroughly chewing each bite.

  - Do not feel compelled to clean your plate. When you feel full, throw your napkin on whatever remains of your meal to discourage you from further nibbling.

These are some simple ideas to help buffer temptations of excess when eating out. As humans, we should expect to fail at times. We will eat too much or make poor choices sometimes. These strategies can help limit those moments. Try them out, see which ones work best for you.

## 4.2.8. Summary

Adopting food habits like these will positively affect hormone levels, metabolic processes, and the microbiome that control and affect weight. Make at most one big change per month and concentrate on developing that as a habit.

To develop good habits, they require a cue, a way to make the habit choice obvious. An example of a habit cue is when you sit down to eat, first enter your food into a calorie tracker. Similarly, recognize the cues of your bad habits. If you always stop at a fast-food establishment on your drive home, maybe avoid the cue (seeing the restaurant) by taking a different route home.[39]

Habits must be made as attractive, something to crave. Restaurants make poor dietary options attractive by using excessive sugar, salt, and fat. It is important to find a way to frame any habit you choose to adopt as some kind of craving. What makes your desired behavior attractive for you?[39]

Make any habit easy to do as a response. Habits require a response to the craving, and this response is more likely to occur if it is easy. Adjust your environment to improve the success of good habits. Place your calorie tracker in the easiest location to access possible. The more times you practice a habit, the more successful you will be. This is true for both good and bad habits. If you eat less added sugars daily by decreasing soda consumption, continuing to do so will get easier. Should you make poor food choice exceptions at fast food establishments, it is easier to continue the poor choice the next time. Concentrate on increasing the frequency of the good habits you decide to adopt.[39]

Lastly, habits result in a satisfying reward. Without a reward, habits will not be sustained. If you avoid eating until after entering the calories of your meal into your calorie tracker, then your reward is the delicious meal. Remove rewards for bad habits. This will make bad habits less attractive. Habit success improves with consistency, repetition, and adjusting your environment.[39]

# 5. Sleep

*"Motivation is what gets you started. Habit is what keeps you going."*

*~Jim Rohn~*

Sleep is critical for good health. Our bodies use sleep to replenish and restore energy. In the United States, 35% of all adults do not sleep enough.[40] Adults require seven hours of sleep or more every night.[41] Many adverse health outcomes are associated with regularly sleeping less than seven hours a night.

These conditions are associated with adults who sleep less than seven hours a night:[40,41]

- Arthritis (18.3% more than those with sufficient sleep)
- Asthma (4.7% more than those with sufficient sleep)
- COPD (3.9% more than those with sufficient sleep)
- Coronary artery disease (1.3% more than those with sufficient sleep)
- Depression (8.3% more than those with sufficient sleep)

- Diabetes (2.5% more than those with sufficient sleep)
- Hypertension
- Heart disease
- Heart attacks (1.4% more than those with sufficient sleep)
- Greater risk of accidents
- Impaired immune function
- Impaired performance
- Increased errors
- Increased pain
- Overall increased risk of death (all-cause mortality)
- Stroke (1.2% more than those with sufficient sleep)
- Weight gain and obesity (Sleeping five hours compared with eight can result in a 3.6% increase in BMI)

Recall that leptin, a hormone secreted by fat cells, functions as a long term signal of positive energy balance. As it rises, the brain recognizes there is sufficient energy storage. Conversely, when leptin levels are decreased, the body considers there to be a need for further energy storage (weight gain). Leptin levels also vary consistently throughout the day in a diurnal manner. At night, leptin levels are highest, which helps us not feel hungry throughout the night.

Studies have demonstrated that sleep restriction reduces leptin levels throughout the day. Leptin is produced during the time spent asleep. This might be the body's way to assure sufficient energy for extended periods of wakefulness during times of sleep restriction.[42]

Ghrelin levels are also affected by changes in sleep. Normally, ghrelin levels are decreased following a meal but then increase again along with increased hunger. The post-dinner rebound occurs in the early part of the night. This rise is interrupted by the onset of sleep. Ghrelin levels then return to the same as those in the morning. Sleep restriction has been shown to result in an overall rise in ghrelin levels within the body.[42]

A hormone called glucagon-like peptide 1 (GLP-1) is produced by cells in the intestines. It acts within the brain in the hypothalamus, promoting the sensation of satiety. It acts concurrently within the gut to slow the emptying of stomach contents contributing to the sensation of fullness. There is some evidence indicating that levels of this hormone are decreased with a lack of sleep. This effect is more pronounced in women and leads to extra weight.[42]

Studies show that when we do not get enough sleep, we eat more. We are hungrier with a larger appetite and often choose less healthy food choices. We have a preference for foods with higher fat content when sleep deprived. Fewer hours of sleep changes the way we view the reward of food. This change in perception of reward with food intake pushes us to choose those unhealthy food choices when we do not have sufficient sleep.

With less sleep, we have more time spent awake. Throughout this time, there is more opportunity to expend energy through physical activity, resting energy expenditure, and the energy of digesting food. Still, sleep restriction has been shown to have no significant effect on our total energy expenditure. There is a tendency towards less energy expenditure! When we do not get enough sleep, the increased calories we consume far outweigh those we burn, ultimately resulting in weight gain.[42]

Studies in those with extra weight who regularly do not sleep enough show that once they do obtain more sleep, there is an association with an overall decrease in appetite and desires for sweet and salty foods.[42]

## 5.1. General Behavioral Strategies to Improve Sleep

The cornerstone of restful and restorative sleep is good sleep hygiene. Sleep hygiene refers to regular sleep habits that promote sleep.

Whenever you struggle with sleep, whether it is falling asleep, staying asleep, or early awakening, revisit this list and modify all you can to promote good sleep:[43]

1. In general, sleep as much as needed to feel refreshed and healthy during the following day, but not more. Curtailing your time in bed will help to solidify sleep. Spending excessively long periods of time in bed is related to fragmented and shallow sleep.

2. Maintain a consistent, regular sleep routine. Begin with setting a routine time to wake up and get out of bed. Wake up at this time every day of the week, including weekends. As your sleep improves, maintain a standard time to go to bed as well. This routine must be maintained every day of the week to obtain restful sleep.

3. Adjust your environment to ensure sleeping success. Ensure you are sleeping in a quiet, dark, relaxing, comfortable environment at a nice temperature. Move the bedroom clock to where you cannot see it, as looking at the clock will keep you awake. Some recommend removing the clock from the bedroom entirely. Remove all screens from the room such as televisions, phones, computers, etc.

4. Prepare for bedtime with a routine. Taking a warm, but not hot, shower one hour before bed can help your body ready for sleep. Consider a light bedtime snack.

Hunger may disturb sleep. Avoid any large meals before bedtime, though.

5. Being physically active during the day can help. More specifically, exercise in the late afternoon or early evening can improve sleep. Avoid exercise within four hours of attempting to go to sleep, as this might keep you awake. Gentle stretching in the evening for relaxation can aid in falling asleep.

6. Do not try to force yourself to sleep. Only go to bed when you feel sleepy. Trying to force yourself to sleep will often make you more awake and is counterproductive. Should you wake up in the middle of the night, let yourself fall asleep within 15-20 minutes. If you cannot fall asleep, get out of bed and sit in the dark in a chair outside your bedroom. Return to bed only when you are sleepy and go to sleep.

7. Use the bed only for sleep and intimacy. Do not watch television, eat, drink, read, have arguments or discussions while in bed. All these activities will work to keep you awake.

8. Avoid napping. Napping interferes with the ability to fall asleep later that night. If you need to nap for safety reasons (driving, etc) then restrict your nap to 30-60 minutes.

9. Avoid coffee, alcohol, and nicotine. Caffeine stays in your body for longer than most people realize and will have effects on your wakefulness. In some people, these effects are more prolonged. Alcohol leads to fragmented sleep and does not provide good restful sleep. Nicotine is a stimulant and reduces the quality of sleep. Additionally, nicotine withdrawal at night will also cause these effects. Quitting smoking and nicotine use is recommended for many health reasons.

10. Should you find yourself struggling to relax your thoughts, keep a notepad and pen close to your bed to write down your thoughts. This is a way for you to note whatever is worrying you allowing you to let it go until morning.

Adopting these sleep habits will enable you to have restful and restorative sleep.

## 5.2. Sleep Restriction Therapy

When people struggle with sleep, they often increase the amount of time in bed trying to sleep but lying awake. Their sleep is fragmented and spread out over many hours. This is not refreshing nor restorative sleep. It is more refreshing to have six hours of sleep in 6.5 hours of time in bed compared with six hours of sleep in nine hours of time spent in bed.

Sleep restriction therapy is a strategy to help people with this struggle. This technique is a way to retrain your body to fall asleep when it is time to sleep. Sleep restriction therapy provides a framework to improve sleep efficiency (the time in bed spent asleep).[43] Know that when starting this process, you may feel more sleepy during the day until your sleep improves. If you experience this increased daytime sleepiness, be mindful of it and take safety cautions as needed.

Here are the steps for sleep restriction therapy:

1. The first step is to maintain a daily sleep log where you track:
   - The time you lie down to go to bed
   - The time you fall asleep
   - The time you wake up to start your day

- When you are asleep and when you are awake at night
- The timing and duration of any naps during the day

2. Calculate your sleep efficiency:
   - Calculate your total sleep time (TST). This is the total number of hours of sleep in a 24-hour timeframe.
   - Calculate your time in bed (TIB). Your time in bed is the total time from when you lie down to fall asleep to the time you get up to start your day. If you take any naps, also include this in the total time.
   - Calculate your sleep efficiency (SE). Sleep efficiency refers to how much of the time spent in bed was spent asleep. This is calculated by dividing the total sleep time by the time in bed and multiplying by 100 for a percentage (TST/TIB x 100).

3. Choose a specific time to wake up every day of the week. Your new total time in bed will be the total time you have spent sleeping (if this is less than six hours, use six hours). Give yourself this amount of time in bed by counting backward from your chosen wake up time.

4. Only make changes to your total time in bed every seven days. Throughout the week, keep track of your sleep efficiency.
   - When your sleep efficiency rises above 90%, increase your time in bed by 15 minutes.
   - Should your sleep efficiency drop below 85%, decrease your time in bed by 30 minutes.

Sleep restriction therapy can be confusing. Here is an example for clarification. Let's say Mary goes to bed at 9 PM, falls asleep at 11 PM, is awake for 1 hour in the middle of the night, and gets out of bed at 6 AM.

Her total sleep time is six hours with a total time in bed of nine hours. This gives her a sleep efficiency of 66% (6/9*100=66%).

Her new time in bed will be six hours as that was her total sleep time. Mary needs to get up at 6 AM for work, so she picks midnight to be her new bedtime. After a couple of weeks of this, she finds she is falling asleep within 15 minutes and sleeping until her wake up time.

Now, her sleep efficiency is 95% (5.75/6*100=95%). She decides to increase her sleep time. Mary moves her bedtime from midnight to 11:45 PM.

In a few weeks and after more adjustments, Mary is going to bed at 10:30 PM, falls asleep within 30 minutes and gets up at 6 AM. Her total sleep time is now seven hours with a total time in bed of 7.5 hours. Her sleep efficiency is 93% (7/7.5*100=93%). She feels like she can sleep better now and is able to maintain this schedule.

## 5.3. Pharmacological Sleep Aids

Several types of medications are used to treat sleep. Medications used to treat insomnia include benzodiazepines, sedative-hypnotics, antidepressants, antihistamines, and those related to melatonin levels.

Benzodiazepines, such as temazepam (Restoril) of traizolam (Halcion), have been used as sleep aids due to their strong sedative effects. They carry concerns of tolerance and dependence. Benzodiazepines have also been associated with other disease processes such as Alzheimer's dementia.

Non-benzodiazepine sedative-hypnotic medications are also indicated for sleep. Zolpidem (Ambien) is the most common sedative-hypnotic in use in the United States. Others are eszopiclone (Lunesta) and zaleplon (Sonata).

Both of these medication classes increase the time of sleep, decrease time to fall asleep, and help people stay asleep. These medications work in the short term and are most useful to help provide a boost initiating good sleep habits for someone with insomnia.

Unfortunately, these can affect how the body metabolizes glucose by decreasing glucose tolerance. Long term use could theoretically lead to weight gain and insulin resistance. Benzodiazepines are habit-forming and can cause withdrawal symptoms if used for more than two weeks. Adverse effects include headaches, nausea, confusion, depression, dizziness, and more.

Some antidepressants are also useful with sleep. A common antidepressant used off-label (not approved by the FDA for insomnia) is trazodone. Its three to six-hour half-life assists those who suffer from falling asleep (sleep onset) and middle insomnia (staying asleep).

Another useful antidepressant class for sleep is the tricyclic acids, which include doxepin and amitriptyline. Doxepin is helpful for sleep maintenance insomnia. Amitriptyline can be helpful in those who wake up early and cannot go back to sleep (late insomnia). The adverse effects of these medications include dry mouth, dizziness, confusion, and unfortunately, weight gain.

Antihistamines are often used as an over-the-counter option to help with sleep. The most common is diphenhydramine (Benadryl or Sominex). Another over-the-counter antihistamine option for sleep is doxylamine (Unisom). While these medications were designed to block histamine, they also limit serotonin re-uptake. This effective increase in serotonin is what provides their sedative properties.

Adverse effects of antihistamine medications include drowsiness, nausea, irritability, dry mouth, urinary retention, rapid heartbeat, and difficulties with concentration. These are not good choices to use for the long term. The longer you use antihistamines, the less effective they become. Insomnia can actually worsen with long term use. Avoid these medications if you have closed-angle glaucoma, heart arrhythmia's, asthma, chronic obstructive pulmonary disease or severe liver disease.

Melatonin is a hormone made by your body that helps maintain your circadian rhythm. Bright light inhibits melatonin, and darkness helps the pineal gland in the brain to release it. When the sun goes down, melatonin rises and lasts for around 12 hours.

Melatonin is classified as a supplement, so is not regulated by the FDA. It can be taken to augment the body's normal melatonin levels.

There is not a lot of quality evidence on melatonin yet, though some promise for its usefulness in sleep onset and middle sleep (awakenings). It appears that melatonin does not help with total sleep, though.

A common dose is 1 mg to 3 mg, which can raise the body's melatonin up to 20 times higher than normal. For best results, it must be taken at the right time of day at an appropriate dosage for the right sleep issue. The typical way to take melatonin is two to three hours before bed. This helps mimic the body's natural level pattern.

A similar medication, ramelteon (Rozerem), works as a melatonin receptor agonist, promoting melatonin effects in the body. It is taken at night about 30 minutes before sleep to boost the effects of melatonin. Unlike other sleep medications, it is not sedating. It is also indicated for long term use when helpful for a person.

Ramelteon is best for problems with sleep onset. In one study, it improved the time to fall asleep by seven minutes compared to placebo and increased the total sleep time by 17 minutes in people with transient insomnia.[44]

Pharmacologic management of sleep problems should most often be viewed as a short term solution only (such as two weeks). The long term usefulness of sleep aids is low. People can develop tolerance and dependence to these medications. Restful sleep is the priority, and while these medications help people fall asleep or stay asleep, they do not provide the restorativeness needed. Use these medications to jump-start new sleep habits.

## 5.4. Some Specific Sleep Conditions

Some sleep conditions are common in those with extra weight such as obstructive sleep apnea (OSA), restless leg syndrome (RLS), and overactive bladder. Managing these conditions effectively contributes to refreshing and restorative sleep.

## 5.4.1. Obstructive Sleep Apnea (OSA)

Obstructive sleep apnea (OSA) is a sleep condition where a person will experience significant airway restriction or complete cessation of airflow during sleep while still trying to breathe. The person will have repeated drops in their blood oxygenation levels and be repeatedly aroused from sleep throughout the night. As those with OSA do not have refreshing sleep, they often also suffer from headaches, excessive daytime tiredness, and higher blood pressure.

OSA is a very common sleep breathing condition. It is estimated that 25% of adults have OSA and up to 45% of those with obesity.[45] These two disease processes are related. Extra weight predisposes a person to develop OSA. More weight also worsens OSA.

Symptoms of OSA include snoring, apneic episodes (moments where the person stops breathing), gasping or choking sensations (that wake the person up), frequent arousals throughout the night, and urinating at night. People with OSA might complain of sore throats, feeling tired, or morning headaches. They might have some mental concerns such as memory or concentration difficulties, daytime tiredness or fatigue, confusion, or mood changes. Common comorbidities associated with OSA are high blood pressure, insulin resistance (diabetes), systemic inflammation, decreased libido, erectile dysfunction, and acid reflux symptoms.

The diagnosis of OSA is made using a sleep study. Scoring severity is described using the apnea-hypopnea index (AHI). This index describes the number of episodes where the person stops or slows their breathing through the night. Normal is less than five episodes at night. Mild OSA is an AHI score between five and 15, moderate from 15 to 30, and severe is any AHI score above 30.

The main treatment modality of OSA is continuous positive airway pressure (CPAP). CPAP is a mild continuous pressure provided through a mask by a small ventilator which helps maintain an open airway for the person throughout the night. There is good evidence that CPAP helps improve the symptoms of OSA and reduce the cardiovascular perils of OSA. Still, many patients find CPAP machines too uncomfortable and decide they prefer to not use their CPAP.

Leptin levels are higher in those with obesity as leptin is directly proportional to the amount of fat. In those who also have OSA, leptin levels are even higher. Besides its important role in satiety, leptin also exerts some control over breathing. After as little as four days of CPAP use, leptin levels decrease.[45] Lower leptin levels let the brain know the body can use up and decrease some energy storage weight.

Levels of adiponectin, another hormone related to obesity and produced in fat cells, are inversely proportional to the amount of fat in the body. Levels are lower in those with a higher BMI. Adiponectin functions to improve the body's metabolism of blood sugar and fatty acids like cholesterol. It also prevents inflammation and atherosclerosis. Regular use of a CPAP machine has been shown to raise adiponectin levels. Higher adiponectin levels encourage the body to lose energy storage weight.

CPAP machines can create a distracting nuisance noise throughout the night. Masks can be uncomfortable to wear and cause other symptoms such as dry mouth. People do not always recognize the improvements from regular use of their CPAP machines on their blood pressure, morning headaches, fatigue, and other symptoms.

Weight loss also helps manage OSA. As people lose weight their OSA improves. For every unit of BMI reduction, there is a corresponding 2.3 unit improvement in AHI score. A 10% loss of weight provides a 20% improvement in OSA severity.[45] Similarly, as a person's OSA is managed with CPAP, they have more restful and refreshing sleep leading to more successful weight loss. In fact, even in those without significant weight loss, the the use of CPAP reduces the amount of fat around their organs (visceral fat)!

As weight loss can improve OSA, a therapeutic role exists for bariatric surgery. Bariatric surgery, discussed in more detail later, can provide significant weight loss helping further improve the severity of OSA.

For successful weight management, in those with extra weight and OSA, it is critical to manage the OSA. Regular use of CPAP cannot be encouraged enough, as this will improve outcomes and assist in weight loss.

## 5.4.2. Restless Leg Syndrome (RLS) and Periodic Limb Movement of Sleep (PLMS)

Restless leg syndrome (RLS) describes an irresistible urge to move your legs. Often, RLS interferes with sleep. It is estimated to affect 7% to 10% of the adult population.[46]

Extra weight increases the risk of RLS. Both of these conditions involve the decreased function of the hormone dopamine in the brain. In those with obesity, there are fewer receptors for dopamine, possibly causing their increased risk for RLS.[47]

RLS is closely associated with periodic limb movement of sleep (PLMS). PLMS describes involuntary limb jerking movements that occur during sleep. Often, these occur every 30 seconds or so. Sometimes these movements will recur throughout the night. Up to 80% of those with RLS will also experience PLMS, though most with PLMS do not have RLS.[46]

Some causes of RLS include iron deficiency anemia, nerve damage (neuropathy), medication side effects (anti-nausea, anti-psychotics, SSRIs, anti-histamines, others), end-stage renal (kidney) disease, and use of alcohol, nicotine, or caffeine.

For those with RLS, appropriate management assists greatly with weight management. Treatment includes avoiding RLS triggers such as alcohol, tobacco, and caffeine. Other helpful therapeutic modalities are compression stockings, leg massage, warm baths, use of heating pads, regular exercise, and leg stretches.[46]

For those with iron deficiency anemia as an underlying cause, iron supplementation is beneficial. Iron supplementation might cause constipation, and if so, can be taken along with a stool softener.

As decreased dopamine activity in the brain is part of the cause of RLS, medications that increase dopamine levels are helpful. Medications that do this are ropinirole (Requip), pramipexole (Mirapex), and rotigotine (Neupro). These medications are very effective for RLS.

Long term use of these medications might lead to worsening of RLS symptoms. When this happens, people experience symptoms earlier in the day or all day long. This seeming progression of the disease process (termed augmentation) is reversed when these medications are discontinued.[46]

Medications such as gabapentin (Neurontin) and pregabalin (Lyrica) have been shown to be effective for moderate to severe RLS. They also help for those with neuropathies and sensory disturbances.

Work closely with your doctor to find the best solution for RLS or PLMS if you suffer from one or both of these syndromes. Work to improve your sleep quality as this will improve your success in your weight journey.

# 6. Stress

*"What consumes your mind controls your life."*

*~Creed~*

When we are stressed, it is easier for us to gain weight. It is more difficult to make healthy dietary choices and our bodies work to retain energy leading us to gain weight. Chronic stress makes it more difficult to lose weight because of these mechanisms.

Stress causes the release of many stress-related hormones. Cortisol, Neuropeptide Y, ghrelin, inflammatory molecules, and serotonin levels all are affected by stress.[48] A state of stress for the body is a state of systemic inflammation. Over time, inflammation results in digestive issues, joint and muscle pains, hypertension, atherosclerosis, and other health issues.

Cortisol, a stress hormone, rises indirectly in response to corticotropin-releasing hormone, which is released in the brain.[48] Cortisol works in response to stress to create a ready energy source for the organs of the body. It increases a person's appetite as well as encourages cravings for foods with fat and sugar. Through its modification of insulin levels and effects, cortisol helps ensure energy availability by increasing the body's fat stores.

Cortisol has many effects on the body. One is to modulate the immune system's inflammatory response. Cortisol reduces the production of some white blood cells (lymphocytes). This might predispose people with obesity or chronic stress to infections. People with increased stress might experience longer times for wounds to heal.

At times of stress, our nerves release a protein named Neuropeptide Y (NPY) in response to higher levels of cortisol and glucocorticoid steroids. NPY is an anxietolytic (reduces anxiety) and functions to modulate stress. This molecule also encourages fat accumulation by unlocking receptors in fat cells, allowing the fat cells to grow in both size and amount. Thus, when stress increases, so does the levels of NPY, which then increase the size of fat cells.

During these times of high stress, we might mindlessly eat. Commonly called stress eating or emotional eating, we snack when we are not hungry. People with high-stress loads tend to snack more, eat fewer meals, and fewer portions of vegetables. Workplace stress is associated with more fast food consumption and mindless eating during tasks.

We often crave comfort foods high in fat and sugar (and calories) when we are stressed. In response to a diet high in fat and sugar, more NPY is released. Foods high in fat and sugar act upon opioid receptors in the brain that help inhibit stress responses. This is partially responsible for a reward circuit when we consume these comfort foods.

Serotonin helps provide the body with a feel-good feeling. Serotonin hormone release is controlled by food intake. Carbohydrate consumption increases serotonin whereas protein intake does not. Because of this effect where carbohydrates increase serotonin levels in the body, people learn to overeat poor food choices, such as potato chips.[49]

Ghrelin, the hunger hormone, also increases in those with chronic stress. As previously discussed, ghrelin encourages increased food consumption. Ghrelin appears to have a role in minimizing the potential for depression behaviors in response to stress. This seems to occur at the expense of our metabolism.[50]

When we are stressed, the combination of ghrelin, plus the effects of increased cortisol, NPY, systemic inflammation, and serotonin push us to consume more, eat more carbohydrates and fats, and increase the size and amount of fat cells in our bodies.

To combat these effects, we must learn to adequately cope with stress. Stress is part of life but should be manageable and intermittent. Let's review general stress management.

## 6.1. Stress Management

Learn to recognize the warning signs of stress. These warning signs manifest themselves as symptoms like anxiety, irritability, or muscle tension. Try to identify whether the stress is justified or exaggerated.

Some level of stress and anxiety should be expected. This is how we stay alive and avoid dangerous scenarios. It is normal to have some level of anxiety in different situations, such as before a speech or an important meeting.

Losing some of your ability to function in daily life is exaggerated stress and anxiety. Being stressed about a potential presentation before an important meeting should not result in avoidance, severe procrastination (which only exacerbates any potential anxiety level), or the development of mindless eating habits.

Accept and welcome the feeling of stress and anxiety when they enable you to improve on performance through increased alertness, perception, and energy. Use the following techniques to reject excessive anxiety and stress when they work against you in your performance or weight management.

There are two general strategies to approach stress management. One approach is to address the stressor directly in an effort to remove or reduce its impact. Alternatively, you can focus on methods that generally reduce the effects of stress, regardless of cause.

## 6.1.1. Directly Address the Causes of Your Stress

To address a stressor directly, you must identify the stressors. One way to do this is to keep a stress diary. For a couple of weeks, record the place and time whenever you feel stressed. Reviewing your notes on your thoughts and your responses to the stressful situations will help provide insight into your stressors and how you react to stress.

Identifying, specifically, what causes stress and anxiety enables you to then purposefully approach each item individually. From this list, rank all the items according to how important they are and how much anxiety or stress they cause. Break these stressors down into what you can do to influence how stressful they are.

For instance, one common and intrusive stressor for people is their financial situation. Much of this is due to uncertainty and a feeling of a lack of control over how much money comes in and how it is spent. Recognizing the stress this situation puts you allows you to approach it head-on.

Making a budget takes effort and time, but budgets reduce much of the stress and anxiety regarding personal finances. A budget helps to provide a sense of control as you remove much of the uncertainty involved. This budget is, in its essence, just a list. You are making a list of all the expected income coming in every month, compared to a list of expenses going out every month. In this way, you gain control and can calmly plan and prepare. You can find places to save money and financially prepare for vacations or gifts so those expenses do not leave you more stressed.

## 6.1.2. General Methods to Reduce Effects of Stress

Here we discuss some general, evidence-backed methods, to reduce stress and anxiety. Some methods to reduce stress include gaining a sense of control, developing an attitude toward stress and anxiety for success, utilizing relaxation techniques, and mindfully investing your energy. Let's discuss those further.

### Gain a Sense of Control

Work to gain a sense of control, similar to how designing a budget can help address the stress of personal finances. Try to plan ahead and allow for sufficient time to get things done. Avoid becoming overwhelmed by your workload by learning to set personal boundaries and learning tactful ways to say "no." These strategies provide psychological comfort from the sensation of control.

Lists help to keep things manageable. They help us to remember things and avoid the worry that we will forget something. They make it easier to prioritize. You can review your lists, identify what is important to do, what can be postponed, delegated, or discarded. This provides an immediate effect on stress and anxiety. Lists provide insights and demonstrate patterns and connections. You can then more strategically find ways to overcome your stressors.

Another way to gain a sense of control is to maintain a clean environment. Clutter can be a physical reminder of mental stressors. Clutter can be more than just physical clutter and can exist in various forms such as mental, emotional, spiritual, or digital. Increased clutter leads to increased stress and anxiety. Look for ways to gain control over clutter as a way to lower your stress and anxiety.

Areas to begin your process of decluttering are those you live in most, such as your bedroom, kitchen, or living room. Similarly, limit the number of tabs you have open in your Internet browser or items saved on your computer desktop. Prioritize decluttering those environments you live in and frequent most.

Removing clutter is important, as is preventing it. Develop habits of putting things away when you finish with them. Avoid incoming digital distractions, making use of do not disturb settings on your smartphone or avoiding reviewing the news or Internet immediately upon awakening.

Use these techniques, regain control of your time, practice saying "no," make lists, declutter, and prevent clutter buildup to gain a sense of control in your life.

### Develop an Attitude Toward Stress and Anxiety for Success

Some of the control over your stress and anxiety is a result of a choice you make, the choice of your attitude. Evidence supports those who are usually optimistic tend to cope better in stressful situations. They also are less likely to become sick compared with those with a more pessimistic outlook. Those with higher optimistic outlooks, compared to those with lower optimistic outlooks, live 14% longer lives.[51]

It is possible to develop a more positive outlook. One way to develop this general optimism is to seek out the positive aspects of situations or events that cause distress. This takes practice and patience. With time it is doable.

When you concentrate on the positive side of a situation, you are less likely to feel negative feelings regarding the situation. You will experience less frustration and hopelessness.

Part of developing a more optimistic attitude is deciding to do so. Seeking the positive aspects of situations requires effort and purpose. It is easy to see the negative aspects of a situation such as an unforeseen detour might. Alternatively, it is much more difficult, but often more rewarding, to find an alternative route that might be helpful in the future to avoid traffic or recognize the beauty in the new scenery the detour offers.

An exercise that helps develop this attitude is to make a daily list of three things you are grateful for or that went well that day. It has been shown that people who perform exercises like this improve their level of happiness, optimism, and physical well-being.

### Relaxation Techniques

Several behaviors promote overall mental and physical relaxation resulting in decreased stress and anxiety. Finding a relaxation technique that works for you will help you to address excessive anxiety and stress.

Relaxation techniques require practice to be effective. Work on activities such as stretching, deep breathing, yoga, meditation, and other relaxation skills as often as you can incorporate into your lifestyle.

Here are a few simple relaxation techniques you can do regularly.

1. Diaphragmatic breathing

One simple relaxation technique is diaphragmatic breathing. Diaphragmatic breathing is another way to describe taking a deep breath by expanding your lungs using your diaphragm muscle. When taking a diaphragmatic breath, your abdomen expands, not your chest. This is our natural and normal way to take a breath. Watch young children breathe for an example to follow. Breathing this way, practicing diaphragmatic breathing, will increase your lung capacity and your body's ability to oxygenate blood.

To perform diaphragmatic breathing, place one hand on your chest and the other on your abdomen. As you take a deep breath, you should feel the hand on your abdomen move out while the hand on your chest remains in place.

This exercise can be done either sitting or standing. Keep your back straight with your feet flat on the floor. Slowly inhale through your nose for four seconds. Now, exhale through your mouth for six seconds. Repeat as desired. Practice diaphragmatic breathing throughout the day.

You might find it helpful in many other situations as well, such as before a presentation or going to bed. Getting adequate sleep can help reduce stress and anxiety.

2. Progressive muscle relaxation

Another relaxation technique is called progressive muscle relaxation. This exercise can be performed either sitting or lying down with your eyes closed. Do this in a quiet location where you can fully relax. Try to be as comfortable as possible, even loosening any restrictive clothing.

If sitting, sit with your arms resting on easily on your lap, palms up, and fingers open and relaxed. Keep your legs uncrossed and feet flat on the floor.

If laying down, have your arms lie next to your body, palms up, in an open relaxed manner. Your feet should be shoulder-width apart.

Take a deep slow breath through your nose using your diaphragm and fill your lungs completely. Slowly breath out through your mouth. Repeat this breathing, taking five seconds to breathe in and five seconds to breath out. Keep breathing in this way until you feel more relaxed or as long as you feel comfortable.

After a few of these breath cycles, move your attention to your toes. Consciously think about each toe and allow each one to fully relax. Then move up through each of your feet. Feel their weight allowing them to sink into the floor or bed. Slowly and consciously move up to your ankles and then calves.

At every point, concentrate on how that part of your body feels. Allow it to relax completely before moving on to the next body part. Continue in this slow and deliberate manner through your entire body. Consciously relax your knees, thighs, hips, buttocks, abdomen, back, and chest. Do not forget to continue to take deep breaths throughout this exercise.

Concentrate on your fingers and hands, again feeling their weight and allowing them to relax fully. Similarly, progress up your arms, shoulders, neck, and head. Progressively relax your face feeling for tension in your jaw, mouth, lips, cheeks, eyebrows, and forehead.

Performing a full-body relaxation exercise takes practice. Should you lose focus, simply return to the last area and continue. You always have the option to return to deep breathing as well.

This is an exercise you can perform daily to reduce stress and anxiety. If able, repeating it twice a day is even better.

## Consider How You Invest Your Energy

Life is too short to spend all your energy into being worried, stressed, or anxious. It is very easy to become overwhelmed by our stressors. A way to reduce our stress and anxiety is to reevaluate how we spend our mental, physical, and emotional energy.

Evaluate those you spend your time with. Spending time with people who are overly critical, negative, or pessimistic can accumulate and manifest in higher stress and anxiety levels for you. You can experience negative psychological consequences when you lack a sense of belonging within a social group. This occurs even in those with a strong social support group. Your choice in friends has consequences for your mental well-being. Spend your time with friends who are positive and refill your mental health tank.

Spend time by investing energy into exercise to lower your stress and anxiety. Exercise helps reduce stress hormones such as cortisol and adrenaline while also promoting the production of endorphins, the feel-good chemicals in the brain. Beneficial exercise can be any activity, from aerobic exercises to resistance exercises.

Try to develop habits incorporating regular physical exercise and activity into daily life. Develop labor-intensive hobbies such as gardening. Go for scheduled walks, runs, or bike rides for good ways to explore your neighborhood and city while being active. Some exercise styles, such as yoga or tai chi, incorporate deep breathing techniques along with low impact movement exercise. These exercises will not only reduce your stress load but also improve your balance and flexibility.

A body of evidence is growing demonstrating an association between social and electronic media use and depression and anxiety.[52,53] There is a dose dependency as well, with more time spent on social media associated with more severe anxiety.[52] Social media provides an illusion of connectivity, increased friendships, and addictive recurrent dopamine surges with likes, comments, and reposts.

Disconnecting or limiting time with social media, either temporarily or permanently, can help lower anxiety levels and improve depression. Here are some ways to limit your social media time:

- Physical strategies:
  - Eliminate all electronics for an hour before going to sleep and after waking up.
  - While working, keep your phone away from you to avoid its distraction.
  - Try to use only one device for logging into social media as opposed to using multiple devices.
- Avoiding the addictive trap of seeing the news-feed:
  - You can turn off all push notifications from social media applications.
  - Subscribe to your favorite websites via email or RSS so that you avoid using social media news-feeds to find their links.
  - When you post on your social media sites, use a third party app so you can avoid seeing the news-feed when you post.

- Protect your time:
  - Restrict yourself to one hour to respond to emails daily.
  - Allow yourself 30 minutes to connect with friends

Interacting with other people on social media is no substitute for interacting with others in real life off of social media. Prioritize investing your energy in being social in real life over time spent on social media. This will lower your stress and anxiety and improve your mental well-being. Some smartphone applications that can help you regain control and limit your social media use listed in Appendix 2.

# 7. Social Aspects of Weight Management

*"The easier it is to do, the harder it is to change."*

*~Eng's Principle~*

There is a strong social component to weight. Your risk of meeting excess weight increases by 37% if your spouse gains weight and meets obesity criteria. If a friend does, your chances to meet obesity criteria increase by 57% to 171%.[54] Some potential explanations for these observations might include sharing eating habits, activity choices, and microbiomes.

In much the same way, successful weight management improves when done as a team. A strong social support network results in a positive impact on stress and anxiety. Supportive friends and family will improve long term success with your weight journey. Working to lose and maintain weight loss with a close friend or family member will improve the success for both of you.

Working and sharing a struggle with someone else brings accountability and company. Work together to remain motivated, keep each other on track, and support each other during shortcomings.

Without evaluating and adjusting your social habits, it will be easy to fall into previous weight traps. Sometimes, the easiest way to avoid overeating a particular food is to avoid any situation where that food is tempting or plentiful. This might mean working within your social circles to eat at new or different establishments. Maybe your best success is to avoid a particular social circle entirely.

When people struggle to stop smoking, they can often identify certain triggers where smoking seems unavoidable, such as when they go bowling. To be successful at smoking cessation, they might face the difficult decision of leaving their bowling league to stop smoking or continue bowling and smoking.

The same is true with losing extra weight. For instance, if it were your habit, you might need to stop meeting for Friday night pizza with work friends if every time you are there, you cannot control the portions of your pizza or other calorie intake. One night of caloric indiscretions can nullify a week of disciplined caloric restriction.

Alcohol can be an easy way to consume more calories than intended. It is a good habit to be on guard for possible moments and situations where you might overindulge in any calorie consuming behavior.

At home, you and your family will eat much more healthy food options when they are the only options available. Having highly processed, calorie-dense foods available only invites poor food choices. Avoid purchasing foods you do not want to eat regularly. This will help you and your family make better food choices when you are hungry and want a quick snack.

# 8. Physical Activity

*"Walking is the best possible exercise.*
*Habituate yourself to walk very far."*

*~Thomas Jefferson~*

Physical activity burns calories. This is the second part of the overly simplified idea of weight management where the difference between the calories we take in, compared to the calories we burn, results in our weight balance.

Exercise can lead to weight loss, but not nearly as much as we often think it does. Compared with the effects of calorie restriction, improving sleep quality, or reducing stress, physical activity only reduces weight by just a fraction.

As already discussed, exercise and physical activity can improve sleep and lower stress and anxiety levels. Exercise and physical activity are critical to long term success with weight loss maintenance and prevention of weight regain after weight loss. This is a strong argument to develop the habit of regular exercise early in your weight journey.

When we gain extra weight, our bodies think this new weight is the weight our body should be. Our bodies then work to maintain this new weight level.

When we lose weight, our bodies make compensating adjustments to help us more easily regain weight. Over time, we might continue to gain weight where at some point our body will change what it considers to be our appropriate weight.

As our bodies lose weight, our lean body mass (non-fat body weight) also decreases. This results in lower energy needs, changes in muscle efficiency during physical activity, and decreases in leptin levels as the fat cells shrink. These changes in our bodies, due to weight loss, work against further weight loss, combating starvation and further weight loss.

The resting and non-resting metabolic rates decrease as you lose weight. This is your body's way of trying to help you maintain what it thinks is your correct weight. Weight loss and the corresponding decrease in lean body mass make it more difficult for further weight loss. Many people are familiar with this weight loss plateau, which is commonly experienced around six months into a weight loss journey.

Overall muscle mass is one driver of the metabolic rate. Muscles require energy to maintain their function. More muscle cells or stronger muscle cells will increase the metabolic rate, increasing the daily caloric needs to maintain weight.

As you lose weight, exercise serves to maintain or buffer the changes in your resting and non-resting metabolic needs. Aerobic exercise, such as walking, jogging, or cycling, is that which utilizes oxygen for respiration and can be done over a long period of time. Resistance exercise, such as weight lifting, is anaerobic exercise.

Aerobic exercise helps consume or burn larger quantities of calories compared to resistance exercise. An adult can estimate a mile to equal about 100 calories. If a person walks or runs three miles, they can roughly estimate they used 300 calories.

Resistance exercise strengthens muscles more than it burns calories at the moment. Resistance exercise can increase the overall metabolic rate burning more calories over the course of the day compared with aerobic exercise.

Exercise will produce a positive impact on leptin and adiponectin levels in the body.[55] Developing a habit of regular exercise allows time for a combination of both aerobic and resistance exercise throughout the week. Aerobic exercise will improve your cardiovascular function and endurance, while resistance exercise will increase muscle mass and your metabolic rate.

When beginning a habit of physical activity and exercise, prioritize activities you enjoy doing. If you enjoy swimming, swim. If it is lifting weights, lift. Make the effort of exercise not something to dread but something to look forward to. Doing so will make physical activity and exercise a successful habit.

Concentrate on the frequency of physical activity before increasing intensity. Before increasing your neighborhood walks from 15 minutes to 30 minutes, work to do them daily. Develop the habit first. Similarly, work on performing resistance exercises more often before increasing how hard you lift.

When losing weight, there is a balancing act as you take in fewer calories than needed to maintain your weight (so you can continue weight loss), yet enough calories to feed muscle growth (to increase your metabolic rate). Too few calories and the body will tap into your muscle cells for energy. Too many calories and the body will store the excess energy in fat cells, undermining your weight loss efforts.

When you exercise, do not consider all the calories burned as extra calories you can consume for that day. We are very bad at estimating how many calories we burn with activities. We are also poor at estimating our intake and portion sizes. To be safe, consider some of those calories as able to be consumed, but not many.

The recommended physical activity time for cardiovascular benefits is 150 minutes of moderate level activity per week. For weight loss, people will often need more than 150 minutes a week combined with calorie restriction. Those who need to prevent weight regain after weight loss might need to participate in more than 300 minutes of moderate level activity every week.[56]

Developing a habit and incorporating the time into your daily routine for physical activity is critical for long term weight management success.

If you currently do not do any extra physical activity, begin with 15 minutes daily. Schedule this time into your day and just go for a walk. Do something easy and rewarding. After successfully incorporating this as a daily activity, then increase the intensity by going for a longer walk or a faster one, whichever you prefer. In this way, you can develop the habit of daily exercise and slowly increase the amount to accommodate your abilities.

Here are some ideas to incorporate more activity and exercise into your daily life:

- At home:
  - Walk, jog, skate, or bicycle.
  - Swim or do water aerobics.
  - Walk your dog.

- While watching television, do stretches, exercises, or pedal a stationary bike.
- Clean your house.
- Wash your car.
- Mow your lawn with a push mower.
- Join an exercise program at work or a nearby gym.
- Take an active class like martial arts, dance, or yoga.
- Join a local walking group.
- Grow a vegetable or flower garden.
- At work:
  - Join a work softball or soccer team.
  - Get off the bus or subway one stop early and walk the rest of the way.
  - Replace a coffee break with a brisk 10-minute walk. See if a friend will go with you.
- Get the whole family involved:
  - Go for an afternoon bike ride with your kids.
  - Push your baby in a stroller.
  - Walk up and down the soccer or softball field sidelines while watching your kids play.
  - Play with your kids – tumble in the leaves, build a snowman, splash in a puddle, or dance to favorite music.

# 9. Medications and Weight Management

*"Success is the sum of small efforts, repeated day in and day out."*

*~Robert J Collier~*

Medications influence your weight, not just those medications used to help lose weight, but also the medications used to treat other medical conditions. Medications can make it easier to lose or gain weight. Before making any decision regarding medications or supplements, discuss the balance of risks and benefits with your doctor.

Medication management as it pertains to weight management is multidimensional. Medicines used to control concurrent disease processes should be optimized to choices that minimize weight gain or encourage weight loss. Medicines specifically indicated for weight loss can be implemented as part of a weight management plan. Supplements can also be considered and discussed.

The decision of how to best manage your health with medications is one you should always make with counsel from your doctor. This section will go over some common medications and some of their characteristics. Because there are often multiple reasons for a particular medicine choice, do not make any changes to your regimen without a conversation where you review the benefits, risks, side effects, and any other alternatives not discussed in this section with your doctor.

## 9.1. Management of Comorbidities

There are many disease processes associated with carrying extra weight. Controlling these comorbidities is critical to living a healthy life and for weight management. Some medicines used to control these associated conditions result in more weight, while alternatives might exist which could be either weight neutral (they do not influence weight significantly in either direction) or weight losing.

The best-case scenario for medical management for all comorbidities is for all your medications to be either weight losing or weight neutral. Often, this is quite difficult to pull off. Minimizing the number of weight gaining medications is a realistic goal. Similarly, finding the lowest effective dose for all medications is also a smart medical move.

Here, we will review some common medical conditions where common weight gaining medication choices can be potentially substituted with a more weight favorable choice. This section is not all-encompassing, and it is wise to review your medication list with your doctor with the specific intent to optimize your overall medical management.

## 9.1.1. Some Select Mental Health Medications

1. **Antidepressants**

   Depression is a common mental health disease process in those with extra weight. Most antidepressants tend to lead to weight gain.

   Selective serotonin re-uptake inhibitors (SSRIs) are a very common class of antidepressants. Examples of SSRIs include sertraline (Zoloft), escitalopram (Lexapro), citalopram (Celexa), fluoxetine (Prozac), and paroxetine (Paxil). All of these can lead to increased weight and sertraline might have the most weight gain of the SSRIs.[57]

   Serotonin-norepinephrine re-uptake inhibitors (SNRIs) are another common antidepressant class. Besides depression, these versatile medications are effective in treating anxiety, some pain syndromes, menopausal symptoms, and other symptoms. Medications included in this class are duloxetine (Cymbalta), venlafaxine (Effexor), and desvenlafaxine (Pristiq). All of these medications can result in increased weight.

   Another class of antidepressant medications that leads to weight gain is the tricyclic acids (TCAs) such as amitriptyline (Elavil) and Nortriptyline (Pamelor). Mirtazapine is in a different antidepressant medication class but also results in weight gain.

   Bupropion (Wellbutrin) acts to inhibit norepinephrine and dopamine re-uptake in the brain. These actions result in its effect as an antidepressant, but it has some other favorable side effects as well. This medication has been found to help with concentration abilities in those who concurrently have some attention deficit hyperactivity disorder tendencies along with depression. Due to its effect on the reward center of the brain, it also helps people with smoking cessation.

Additionally, given how it affects dopamine and norepinephrine in the hypothalamus within the brain, bupropion leads to appetite suppression and satiety. Thus, this antidepressant is associated with weight loss.

For those who meet the weight criteria for overweight or obesity and are depressed, bupropion is a reasonable first choice. For those who respond best to SSRIs, an SSRI to consider with the least associated weight gain is fluoxetine (Prozac).[57]

One common eating disorder is night eating syndrome. In this syndrome, people tend to crave and consume a high level of carbohydrates in the evenings while not eating in the mornings. They might even wake up at night hungry and eat. For those with night eating syndrome, sertraline is effective.[58] This is an example of a case where a medication with weight gaining tendencies can instead be useful to help a person lose weight.

2. **Antipsychotics**

Antipsychotic medications are prescribed for many mental health disorders and often cause weight gain. This weight gain can be significant depending on the agent. Antipsychotics are a difficult class of medications to optimize as once the person is stable on one of these medications, it is best to not make changes. Similarly, when making changes, these medications usually should be adjusted gradually, and not all antipsychotics work in the same way for every person.

Any medication adjustment must be made cautiously and carefully.

The antipsychotic medications associated with the most weight gain are clozapine (Clozaril) and olanzapine (Zyprexa). Each is associated with over a 4 Kg (8.8 lbs) weight gain. Risperidone (Risperdal) is also associated with weight gain, though less than 4 Kg.

While also associated with weight gain, alternative antipsychotic medication options associated with less weight gain to consider are ziprasidone (Geodon), aripiprazole (Abilify), and haloperidol (Haldol).

Should you find yourself requiring one of these medications and want to consider a change, coordinate with both your primary care doctor (PCP) and psychiatrist. Your PCP can communicate your hopes and goals with your psychiatrist to find a more weight centric alternative if possible. Together, they can help determine the balance of the risks of any change to your regimen compared with the potential benefits.

3. **Stimulants**

Stimulants are commonly used to treat attention deficit hyperactivity disorder. Medications such as amphetamine/dextroamphetamine (Adderall), methylphenidate (Concerta), or lisdexamfetamine (Vyvanse) all share the side effect of appetite suppression where the person might forget to eat. Everyone (especially children) who is taking a stimulant should be weighed regularly to assure appropriate weight (or growth in children).

One of these stimulants, lisdexamfetamine, has been approved for moderate to severe binge eating disorder. This drug increases the dopamine and norepinephrine levels in the hypothalamus within the brain. This results in decreasing appetite and increasing satiety. Lisdexamfetamine helps with compulsion control, craving control, and impulsivity control.

These medications carry a concern of abuse, dependence, and tolerability. For these concerns, they are all controlled substances. Stimulants should only be used for specific indications and the decision to initiate or continue therapy with one of these agents should be made with open communication with your doctor.

# 9.1.2. Some Select Endocrine Medications

1. **Diabetes Mellitus**

   Diabetes is a very common endocrine disease where the body cannot regulate blood sugar (glucose) levels effectively. Insulin is either insufficiently produced or the body becomes less responsive to insulin's effects. Those with extra weight and associated diabetes typically have diabetes mellitus type 2, meaning their bodies are resistant to insulin. Insulin is released after a rise in blood glucose, but the body's mechanisms to control the glucose level are dampened.

   The most important medication for someone with diabetes type 2 is metformin (Glucophage). Metformin works to decrease glucose production in the liver, decrease the absorption of sugar in the gastrointestinal tract, and increase the sensitivity of insulin in cells around the body. Metformin helps the body respond to glucose intake in a more normal fashion resulting in less total insulin.

   As discussed earlier, insulin is a hormone that promotes weight gain. When on metformin, there is less total insulin exposure, so metformin is weight neutral in some and weight losing in others. Additionally, metformin has been demonstrated to reduce all-cause mortality and diseases of aging.[59] It is currently recommended as first-line treatment for diabetes right after lifestyle modification.[60]

   Two medication classes commonly used to treat diabetes are sulfonylureas like glimepiride (Amaryl) or glipizide (Glucotrol), and the thiazolidinediones (TZDs) such as pioglitazone (Actos) and rosiglitazone (Avandia). These medications are often chosen for use in diabetes for their price, as the generic versions are very affordable. They have been recommended, until recently, early in the treatment algorithm for diabetes as they were not expensive and they improved diabetes lab values. Unfortunately, they also result in extra weight.

With the sulfonylureas, people tend to gain over 4 Kg (8.8 lbs) of weight. With TZDs, people can expect to gain a little less compared to the sulfonylureas. Sulfonylureas work by increasing the pancreatic release of insulin within the body. The stimulated insulin is released in response to the medication and not in relationship to food. These medications result in higher total insulin exposure along with their expected weight gain.

There are some newer medications useful in managing diabetes which result in weight loss. Evidence is growing in support of the use of these medications earlier in diabetes management. One drawback for their use is their expense, though this has been improving. These medications are preferable to the sulfonylureas and TZDs for several reasons but are sometimes limited by their price-tag.

Those with diabetes have an inappropriate insulin response to food intake than those without diabetes. This is partially due to the function of hormones called incretins. Incretins are hormones that stimulate insulin release from the pancreas in response to food intake. One important incretin is called glucagon-like peptide-1 (GLP-1).

GLP-1 is produced in the small intestine and stimulates insulin release only when there is glucose in the bloodstream. Within the gastrointestinal tract, it acts to delay stomach emptying which results in slower absorption of carbohydrates and a slower rise in blood glucose levels with meals. GLP-1 also acts within the hypothalamus in the brain to curb appetite and lead to satiety.

GLP-1 agonists are medications that mimic incretin activity. These include exenatide (Byetta), liraglutide (Victoza), dulaglutide (Trulicity), and Lixisenatide (Adlyxin). These medications are injected but are not insulin. They help the body more appropriately secrete insulin when it is needed (elevated blood glucose). Besides improved diabetes control, their actions result in less overall total insulin exposure and thus weight loss.

Dipeptidyl peptidase-IV (DPP-4) is an enzyme that inactivates the activity of incretins. Medications that inhibit this enzyme, DPP-4 inhibitors, allow for the incretins your body produces to act for a longer period of time. Thus, they function similarly to the GLP-1 agonists, though indirectly and less intensely.

Some examples of DPP-4 inhibitors are sitagliptin (Januvia), saxagliptin (Onglyza), and alogliptin (Nesina). These medications slow the inactivation of incretin hormones. Their actions result in improved blood glucose control, insulin secretory response, and insulin sensitivity. For the same reasons as with the GLP-1 agonists, they are associated with weight loss, though not as strongly. These medications are less expensive than the GLP-1 agonists and not injected.

The kidneys filter the blood to remove waste products. As they filter the blood, the kidneys initially filter out glucose, then later reabsorb the glucose up to a certain point. Any glucose that remains above that point ends up excreted in the urine. In normal circumstances, this cut-off point is high enough that all glucose is reabsorbed. For those with diabetes and high blood glucose, the kidneys cannot reabsorb all the glucose initially filtered out.

The reabsorption process of glucose in the kidneys requires a protein called the sodium/glucose cotransporter 2 (SGLT2). This protein can be inhibited by medications like canagliflozin (Invocana), dapagliflozin (Farxiga), ertugliflozin (Steglatro), and empagliflozin (Jardiance). When the reabsorption process is interrupted with this class of medications, the person will urinate out excess glucose, lowering the overall glucose load in their body. This helps to improve their glucose control but has also been shown to improve blood pressure and result in weight loss. Use of SGLT2 medications is associated with an average 3 Kg weight loss.[61]

At some point, most people with diabetes will require insulin. Many types of insulin can be used in the management of diabetes. There are short-acting insulins, intermediate-acting insulins, insulins that last all day long, and mixes of multiple duration insulins.

As already covered, increased total insulin exposure results in extra weight. The goal with insulin management, then, is to use as little as needed. One weight-conscious strategy is to use long-acting insulin, at as low a dose as needed, for diabetes control in combination with other modalities.

In summary, for those with extra weight and diabetes, avoid the sulfonylurea and TZD classes. If possible, use a GLP-1 agonist (or DPP-4 inhibitor) and an SGLT2 inhibitor. If insulin is required for diabetes control, preference should be made for longer-acting insulin used once a day (compared with twice a day). Metformin is recommended for all patients with diabetes who do not have a contraindication.

2. **Thyroid Disease**

The thyroid hormones help regulate the body's overall metabolic rate. Too little thyroid hormone and people experience fatigue, weakness, thinning hair, depression, constipation, memory issues, joint pain, and weight gain. Symptoms of too much thyroid hormone include nervousness, restlessness, difficulty with concentration, irregular or fast heartbeat, hair loss, nausea and vomiting, and possibly weight loss.

Hypothyroidism is treated with a medication called levothyroxine (Synthroid). This is a synthetic version of the thyroid hormone.

The brain releases thyroid-stimulating hormone (TSH) in response to thyroid hormones (T3/T4). The TSH level is used to monitor the therapeutic dosing levels of levothyroxine. When the TSH is elevated, the brain is trying to stimulate the thyroid to release more hormones. A higher dose of levothyroxine is needed.

Over-treatment can lead to dangerous arrhythmia's and bone loss with fractures. When the TSH level is below normal, the levothyroxine dose should be decreased.

For those with extra weight and hypothyroidism, levothyroxine dosing should be adjusted so the TSH levels are within the normal range, potentially favoring the lower end of that range. As always, the risks and benefits are individualized and it is recommended to have this discussion with your doctor.

3. **Steroid Medications**

Systemic corticosteroids such as prednisone, are helpful in the management of asthma to rheumatic disorders. These medications modulate cortisol in the brain. Cortisol, just as when stressed, exerts its effect on the hypothalamus resulting in increased appetite, food cravings, and changes in overall metabolism.

Systemic corticosteroids are similarly associated with weight gain. Their effects are more pronounced the longer and more regular a person uses corticosteroids. These medications also carry other risks including bone loss, diabetes, psychiatric disturbances, and more.

In general, and especially for those with extra weight, it is recommended to limit your total exposure to corticosteroids as much as practical. As far as you are able to, use the lowest dose needed or avoid these medications altogether.

There are some medical disease states for which a person relies on corticosteroids to help manage and control their symptoms. In those situations, it might be impossible to avoid using corticosteroids.

Topical steroids and steroid joint injections are not associated with the weight gain discussed here.

4. **Contraception Medications**

There are many types of hormonal contraception medications. These medications are molecules that function in the body in a similar fashion as either progesterone hormone or estrogen hormone.

All hormonal contraception medications consist of a progesterone medication with or without an estrogen medication. The individual components and their dosages are designed to take advantage of certain effects. For instance, some oral contraceptive pills (OCPs) are also approved to treat acne.

OCPs historically contained much higher doses of their individual components. Estrogen can increase appetite and promote water retention. Most combinations today contain much lower doses of estrogen than years ago, where remain effective for birth control but are much less likely to promote weight gain.

Today, if a woman gains weight after initiating an OCP, it is most likely water retention and not fat accumulation.

Women who use a progesterone-only pill might gain less than 2 Kg (4.4 lbs) after six to 12 months of use. This weight often resolves when she stops taking the progesterone-only pill.[62]

Other forms of hormonal contraception include medroxyprogesterone injection (Depo-Provera), levonorgestrel intrauterine device (Mirena, Skyla), and etonogestrel (Nexplanon).

With the levonorgestrel intrauterine devices, only a few (5%) of women experience weight gain. Studies comparing body composition changes after 12 months of progesterone device use (including levonorgestrel and etonogestrel) do not indicate a change compared with devices without progesterone.[63] Weight gain after 12 months was less than 2 Kg (4.4 lbs).[64]

Medroxyprogesterone, an injection received every three months, is associated with over 4 Kg (8.8 lbs) of weight gain. Avoid choosing this contraception option if you struggle with weight.

## 9.1.3. Some Select Cardiovascular Medications

Medications to control blood pressure that increase weight include amlodipine (Norvasc), nifedipine (Procardia), and beta-blockers.

Amlodipine and nifedipine are in a class of medication called calcium channel blockers. These can cause some water retention and swelling. This increased weight is not from fat storage.

Beta-blocker medications are associated with a weight gain of about 1.2 Kg (2.6 lbs). Medication examples from this category are atenolol (Tenormin), metoprolol (Lopressor), and propranolol (Inderal).

It is not clear why these beta-blocker medications are associated with weight gain. They do limit the heart rate and might decrease exercise tolerance and overall activity levels. They might also slow metabolism. Newer beta-blockers, such as carvedilol (Coreg) are less likely to cause weight gain.

# 9.1.4. Some Select Neurology Medications

Common neurological medications that result in weight gain are those that control seizures (antiepileptics). Medications to control seizures that might increase weight include carbamazepine (Tegretol), gabapentin (Neurontin), and valproic acid (Depakene). Alternative medication choices with less associated weight gain are zonisamide (Zonegran), topiramate (Topamax), lamotrigine (Lamictal), and levetiracetam (Keppra).

Zonisamide is an antiepileptic used to treat partial seizures. Some patients lose weight while on zonisamide. In conjunction with a reduced-calorie diet, zonisamide results in an additional average of 5 Kg (11 lbs) of weight loss compared with diet alone.[65] For this reason, it has also been used off label for weight loss.

Another antiepileptic medication, topiramate, is used for partial and generalized seizures. It is also indicated for migraine headache prophylaxis decreasing the headache frequency. Many people lose weight while taking topiramate. It is now also approved as part of a combination medication for obesity which will be discussed later.

97

Lamotrigine and levetiracetam are considered weight neutral medications but have been shown to result in a significant weight loss in some individuals. Levetiracetam is indicated to treat partial and generalized seizures. In post-marketing reports, it was found this medication helps with weight loss. Lamotrigine is indicated for bipolar disorder in addition to partial and generalized seizures.

In general, when possible, avoid valproic acid (50% of people will gain weight).[66] For those with extra weight and seizure disorders, preference is placed on topiramate, zonisamide, levetiracetam, and lamotrigine. For those with extra weight and chronic migraine headaches, topiramate might be a good choice to lower their frequency and intensity. For those with bipolar disorder, lamotrigine might be worth consideration.

None of these medications should be stopped abruptly. Any medication change must be made in a partnership with your doctor.

## 9.2. Medications for Weight Loss

Historically, we have struggled to find good medications for weight loss. Medications might result in weight loss, but also with severe adverse reactions. We now know that part of this difficulty in finding effective weight loss agents is due to the broad spectrum of disease process that obesity entails. Much of obesity is hormonally regulated, and more recent medications developed for weight loss attempt to address these aspects of the disease process.

Currently, several medications are indicated for weight loss that can only be used for the short term (less than three months). Newer agents are approved for long term use. They can be used indefinitely, with support from studies lasting up to two years in duration.

Long term medications are preferable as obesity is a chronic disease process, similar to hypertension. Just as it would be illogical to treat high blood pressure to a controlled level with a medication for three months and then stop medications when the person's blood pressure was at goal, it is illogical to treat extra weight until a person reaches a goal weight and then stop treatment.

Medications for weight loss are indicated in those with a BMI over 27 Kg/m$^2$ who also have a weight-related comorbidity such as high blood pressure, high cholesterol, diabetes mellitus, or obstructive sleep apnea. They are also indicated for anyone with a BMI of over 30 Kg/m$^2$. None are indicated for use during pregnancy.

## 9.2.1. Short Term Weight Loss Medications

The low cost of the short term medications in weight management provides much of their usefulness and popularity. Their usefulness is hampered by potentially serious adverse effects.

Medications to use for just a few weeks (short term) for weight loss are phentermine (Adipex), diethylpropion (Tenuate), and phendimetrazine (Bontril). These medications function similarly to amphetamine resulting in appetite suppression. It is thought that they stimulate the hypothalamus in the brain to release norepinephrine, causing a reduction in appetite. Expected weight loss with these medications is between 2% and 6% of body weight.

All of these medications are controlled substances and carry the potential for dependence, tolerance, and addiction. Common adverse effects include dry mouth, insomnia, dizziness, palpitations, increased blood pressure, irritability, and more. Severe adverse effects include heart valve disorders, elevated pulmonary pressure, and psychotic disorder.

The limited-time duration of use for these medications by the FDA is due to the paucity of studies demonstrating long term efficacy and safety. Still, there is some evidence for long term effectiveness and safety. Diethylpropion has demonstrated sustained weight loss past 1 year with no increased rates of cardiovascular or psychiatric disease.[67] Phentermine is approved as part of a combination long term weight loss medication, though in a lower dose than commonly prescribed when by itself.

The best candidates for these medications might be younger patients who need short term assistance with appetite suppression. Those with uncontrolled blood pressure, coronary artery disease, hyperthyroidism, glaucoma, anxiety, insomnia, or a history of drug abuse should not use these medications.

## 9.2.2. Long term Weight Loss Medications

Effective weight management medications that can safely be used longer than 12 weeks are a relatively recent development in medicine. These medications can be characterized as fat blockers, stimulants, antidepressants, or diabetes medications.[68] The long term weight management medications are orlistat (Xenical/Alli), lorcaserin, naltrexone/bupropion, liraglutide, and phentermine/topiramate. There are specific therapeutic benefits and adverse effects with each of these medications.

1. **Orlistat (Xenical/Alli)**

   Orlistat has been approved by the FDA and used for several years. It works by reducing the absorption of fats from food through inactivation of gastric (stomach) and pancreatic fat specific enzymes (lipases).

This medication is modestly effective with an average of 2.5 to 3.4 Kg (5.5 to 7.5 lbs) weight loss. There is both an over-the-counter dose and a prescription dose of this medication. It is recommended to consume a diet of less than 30% fat and to take orlistat with every meal.

The adverse effects of orlistat include increased gas, abdominal cramps, oily stools, and sometimes even fecal leakage. These are worsened when the diet is higher in fats. Unfortunately, its effectiveness on weight is also increased with more fat in the diet. Due to the adverse effects, orlistat is not typically well-tolerated and many people prefer to use a different medication.

Despite these effects, though, orlistat (as Alli) is the only weight management medication available over-the-counter (OTC). With the OTC formulation available for around $50, it is one of the more affordable long term weight medications.

2. **Lorcaserin (Belviq)**

Lorcaserin stimulates the 5-hydroxytryptophan 2c receptors (serotonin) in the hypothalamus of the brain. These, in turn, activate the anorexigenic pathway. Activation of this pathway results in decreased food intake due to decreased appetite, satiety, and an increased sense of fullness.

The FDA has approved lorcaserin as a long term weight management medication. It is indicated to augment a reduced-calorie diet and exercise in a chronic weight management program for those with a BMI above 30 Kg/m$^2$ or those with a BMI above 27 Kg/m$^2$ with a weight-related comorbidity such as high blood pressure, type 2 diabetes, or high cholesterol.

This medication is modestly effective and well-tolerated. The average weight loss associated with lorcaserin is 2.9 to 3.6 Kg (6.4 to 7.9 lbs). Common adverse effects include headaches, dizziness, fatigue, dry mouth, constipation, and upper respiratory illnesses.

As lorcaserin modulates the serotonin receptors in the hypothalamus within the brain, those taking an SSRI antidepressant should not use this medication. Those with migraines should also avoid taking lorcaserin. There is a concern for the development of cardiac valvular disease, so this medication is not a good choice for those with a heart murmur.

For people with inadequate meal satiety, lorcaserin can be a good option.

3. **Bupropion/Naltrexone (Contrave)**

This long term weight loss medication is a combination of two other medications, bupropion and naltrexone. Bupropion, a dopamine and norepinephrine re-uptake inhibitor, increases the levels of those hormones within the hypothalamus of the brain stimulating the anorexigenic (satiety) pathway. Naltrexone is an opioid receptor antagonist, meaning it blocks the opioid receptors. This acts on the proopiomelanocortin (POMC) neurons in the hypothalamus to curb appetite.

Together, these medications decrease appetite and regulate the dopamine reward system in the brain. This helps to control food cravings and overeating behaviors. The average weight loss for people on this medication is 3.7 to 5.2 Kg (8.15 to 11.46 lbs).

During the first few months on this medication, a person's blood pressure might increase. Other adverse effects include nausea, constipation, headaches, vomiting, dizziness, insomnia, and dry mouth. Nausea is particularly common. It is contraindicated for those with uncontrolled hypertension, those with a history of seizures, or with long term opioid use.

People who experience cravings for food, or addictive behaviors related to food, benefit from this combination. As bupropion is an antidepressant and also helps people stop smoking, it can be a good choice for those with concomitant depression or who are trying to quit smoking. Because of naltrexone, this combination also helps those who drink alcohol to reduce their intake.

4. **Liraglutide (Saxenda)**

Liraglutide is a GLP-1 agonist and is used to treat diabetes as described earlier. There are GLP-1 receptors both in the gastrointestinal (GI) tract as well as in the hypothalamus in the brain. The receptors in the GI tract slow the emptying of the stomach, increasing the feeling of fullness. The GLP-1 receptors in the brain affect appetite regulation.

The liraglutide dose for weight management is twice that of the dose to treat diabetes (3mg daily instead of 1.2mg daily). This medication is delivered via injection. The average weight loss associated with liraglutide is 5.8 to 5.9 Kg (12.79 to 13 lbs).

Adverse effects include nausea, diarrhea, vomiting, constipation, heartburn, and abdominal pain. Those with a history of pancreatitis should not use liraglutide. Similarly, those with a personal or family history of medullary thyroid cancer or multiple endocrine neoplasia syndrome type 2 should not either. People afraid of needles are not good candidates.

This is a good medication for people who have extra weight and impaired glucose tolerance, pre-diabetes, or diabetes type 2. For those who also require psychiatric medications, liraglutide is a good option.

## 5. **Phentermine/Topiramate (Qsymia)**

The combination of phentermine and topiramate is the most effective medication currently available for weight loss. It is associated with an average weight loss of 4.1 to 10.7 Kg (9 to 23.59 lbs).

Phentermine is an adrenergic agonist, a stimulant, that works in the hypothalamus of the brain through norepinephrine to decrease appetite and improve satiety. Phentermine targets dopamine and norepinephrine, which work together to increase leptin levels in the bloodstream. This increased leptin tells the brain that the body does not need more energy storage, leading to appetite suppression.

Topiramate is a neurostabilizer that enhances the activity of gamma-aminobutyric acid (GABA) in the brain. This also results in an increased feeling of fullness and even some prevention of fat absorption. Topiramate has an adverse effect of making foods taste less appealing, which also likely contributes to the decreased appetite.

Adverse effects include increased heart rate, birth defects (cleft palates associated with the topiramate), insomnia, dizziness, constipation, dry mouth, and abnormal skin sensations (paresthesias). People with uncontrolled blood pressure, heart disease, sensitivity to stimulants, or a history of drug abuse should not use this medication. Other conditions that a person might have and should avoid this medication include hyperthyroidism, glaucoma, anxiety, insomnia, and a history of kidney stones.

Good candidates to use phentermine and topiramate are younger patients who need assistance with appetite suppression.

6. **Summary**

All of these medications, when used for a year and compared with placebo, are associated with achieving the clinically meaningful weight loss goal of 5% to 10% of their weight. Phentermine-topiramate and liraglutide carry the highest odds of achieving the 5% weight loss.

Here is a ranking of these long term weight loss medications in terms of most weight loss to least:

1. Phentermine-topiramate
2. Liraglutide
3. Naltrexone-bupropion
4. Lorcaserin
5. Orlistat
6. Placebo

The positive effects on weight are counterbalanced by discontinuation rates due to the adverse effects people might experience. Here are the same medications ranked by their rate of discontinuation due to their adverse effects:

1. Placebo
2. Lorcaserin
3. Orlistat
4. Phentermine-topiramate
5. Naltrexone-bupropion
6. Liraglutide

The best long term weight loss medication choice for you is the one you can safely tolerate and is effective to meet your goals. This decision is one you make shared with your doctor. As the research and body of understanding increases regarding how weight homeostasis is regulated, we can expect to continue to see effective and safer long term weight loss medication options developed and produced in the future.

## 9.3. Supplements and Over-the-Counter Options for Weight Loss

People often desire other over-the-counter options in the form of supplements to aid in their weight management. Evidence to support their effectiveness and safety is often lacking or exceedingly weak and overall they need more studies before strong recommendations can be made.

## 9.3.1. Functional Foods

Dietary fiber was discussed earlier with food intake. As a functional food, it is thought to increase satiety and lead to weight reduction and waist circumference reduction. Fiber delays the digestion and absorption of carbohydrates, lessening insulin spike peaks, and attenuating the growth in the size of fat cells. Soluble fiber, such as that found in oats, legumes, and barley, may reduce fatty liver, improve cholesterol levels, and increase sensitivity to insulin.[69]

Prebiotics are indigestible compounds called oligosaccharides that are thought to stimulate bacterial growth in the intestines. The bacteria thought to be most affected are the lactobacilli and bifidobacteria in the colon. Probiotics are bacteria such as lactobacilli which protect against yeast and pathogenic bacteria. The use of prebiotics and probiotics affects fat metabolism through effects on the intestinal nervous system signaling, calorie absorption from the diet, and immune system signaling. They can help adjust bacterial flora to lean more towards lactobacillus and bifidobacterium instead of bacteroidetes, which aids in weight management.[69]

Other potentially beneficial functional foods are monounsaturated fatty acids (found in olive oil, canola oil, avocados, nuts, and seeds) and polyunsaturated fatty acids (found in vegetable oils, nuts, and seeds). Consuming saturated fats leads to an increased size of fat cells. When unsaturated fats are substituted for saturated fats, they result in lipolysis (breaking up of fat cells), lower inflammation, and improved dyslipidemia.[69]

Phenols have beneficial effects on weight as well. These are found in coffee and teas as caffeic acid, capsaicin from chili peppers, curcumin (curry) from turmeric, and even propolis made by bees from resin in trees. Curcumin might reduce body fat by reducing the making of fat (lipogenesis), as well as improve the metabolic function of the fat cells, immune function, and metabolic disease.[69,70]

Onions and garlic contain thiols and sulfides. Garlic improves cholesterol and blood sugar metabolism, though it is unclear if it affects fat cells themselves. In some animal studies, onion extract reduced body weight and lowered glucose levels.[69]

Phytoestrogens, found in nuts, flax-seeds, soybeans, and soy products, might reduce abdominal fat and cholesterol levels. They potentially could improve the metabolism of blood sugar as well.[69]

## 9.3.2. Supplements

There are many supplements available for purchase to aid in weight loss. These are sold individually or as part of a formulation. It is wise to use caution with any supplement use, as these often have not been evaluated for safety. For instance, one of the most popular weight loss supplements, Hydroxycut made by Iovate Health Sciences, has lead to the death of multiple people, and removed from the market twice. After each removal, it returned to the market in a reformulated manner.[71]

Bitter Orange (citrus aurantium) is an extract of the bitter orange peel and contains synephrine alkaloids. These potentially increase satiety due to structural and functional similarities to ephedrine. Just as ephedra, which was banned, bitter orange can result in higher blood pressure and risk of cardiovascular events like a heart attack.[69,72]

*Garcinia cambogia* is a fruit native to India that contains an acid (hydroxycitric acid) that increases satiety, possibly the metabolic rate, and decreases fat storage in adipocytes. It may cause short term weight loss and is well-tolerated, but might result in increased liver enzymes and damage.[69,72]

Hoodia comes from a spiny succulent plant from South Africa. Its flowers smell like rotten meat and are pollinated by flies. The indigenous people have used Hoodia to reduce their appetites on long hunting trips. Hoodia increases satiety through its effect within the hypothalamus. Hoodia may promote weight loss, but it also can result in high blood pressure, elevated heart rate, and increases in bilirubin and a liver enzyme called alkaline phosphatase.[69]

Glucomannan and guar gum, are ground into a powder and used as weight loss supplements. When mixed with water, they become a thick, viscous mixture that could block the intestinal absorption of fats and increase satiety.[69] Evidence to support the effectiveness of these supplements remains weak.[72]

African mango seeds, *Irvingia gabonensis*, may result in increased satiety, lower levels of leptin, and increased levels of adiponectin. These changes in hormone levels and satiety lower body weight, improve cholesterol levels and can reduce inflammatory markers.[69] Common adverse effects include headache, flatulence, and insomnia. While data on its effectiveness appears encouraging, it is not recommended.[73]

Chitosan is a supplement that is made from the exoskeletons of crustaceans and arthropods. It slows down the absorption of fat within the intestinal tract, lowering body weight, and decreasing fat. It could result in lower blood sugar and triglyceride levels.[69] Evidence on the effectiveness of chitosan is limited but is possibly effective. It should be avoided in those with a shellfish allergy.[72,73]

Pyruvate theoretically increases metabolism at the cellular level resulting in improvement of exercise endurance. This theoretically would result in increased energy expenditure and thus, weight reduction and improved adipocyte cell function.[69] Pyruvate is well tolerated and possibly beneficial for weight loss.[73]

Carnitine is an amino acid that helps the mitochondria (the energy producer) within cells. It increases the breaking down of fats in adipocyte cells shrinking the size of the fat cells and their triglyceride levels. As it might also attenuate the effects of anaerobic training and cell damage, taking carnitine could result in greater energy expenditure and help with fat weight reduction.[69]

Collagen hydrolysate, digestible proteins from bones and cartilage, might increase thermogenesis and reduce inflammatory markers. If the collagen helps with joint mobility, its use could facilitate energy expenditure with increased activity.[69] The actual effectiveness is uncertain.

## 9.3.3. Minerals and Vitamins

Chromium is an essential element used in the body for carbohydrate and lipid metabolism. Supplementation with chromium in those with diabetes type 2 might result in weight loss, improved insulin sensitivity, and glucose control.[69] Still, chromium has uncertain efficacy in humans for weight loss.[72]

Manganese might be helpful to supplement if you are deficient.

There is little evidence that zinc supplementation might improve weight or metabolic disease.[69]

Studies regarding calcium and weight loss vary widely. When on a calorie-restricted diet, substituting calcium-enriched foods for less healthy foods might augment fat weight loss, improve fat function, and improve metabolic disease. Some animal studies indicate calcium increases thermogenesis, increases adipocyte lipolysis, and decreases body weight.[69]

Vitamin D levels tend to be lower in those with extra weight. Vitamin D deficiency does not cause weight gain, but weight gain results in a deficiency of vitamin D. This happens because the fat-soluble vitamin is diluted within the increased fat stores. Also, people with extra weight often wear extra clothing blocking from sunlight and spend less leisure time spent outdoors. Low vitamin D results in increased parathyroid hormone, as the body attempts to increase the vitamin D levels. When taking combined calcium and vitamin D, this will normalize the body's attempts to raise its levels, reducing the calcium levels inside the adipocytes. This, in turn, up-regulates lipid (fat) utilization through decreasing lipogenesis (making of new fats), increasing fat oxidation (usage) rates, and increasing diet-induced thermogenesis. These changes reduce spontaneous calorie intake culminating in weight reduction.[69]

Vitamin B12 (cyanocobalamin) deficiency is associated with extra weight.[74] Supplementing B12 when a person is deficient might help with weight loss. B12 helps contrib-

110

ute to weight loss by assisting in the metabolism of lipids and protein, providing more energy. In the body, vitamin B12 helps to produce serotonin which improves overall feel-good sensation and can help with satiety. Despite these theoretical expectations, its real effect on weight loss remains uncertain.

# 10. Bariatric Surgery

*"Our greatest battles are that with our own minds."*

*~Jameson Frank~*

Bariatric surgery is often thought of as a procedure of last resort. Some avoid making the choice of surgery, stating it feels like a sign of failure in some way. Neither of these thoughts is accurate; surgery should not be a procedure of last resort and it does not reflect personal failure.

Surgery should be considered objectively as part of a weight loss and weight management strategy. Research has demonstrated positive outcomes in regards to these procedures.

People lose more weight with bariatric surgery compared with nonsurgical weight loss interventions. In the short term, people can lose 60% to 70% of their extra weight and maintain a 50% loss of their extra weight 10 years later.[75]

Weight loss surgery is also associated with reductions in all-cause mortality of 30% to 50% after seven to 15 years. In those with diabetes, remission occurs in 60% to 80% of patients after the roux-en-Y surgery procedure.

This remission is retained for up to 15 years in 30% of patients.[75]

More often than not, surgery is discussed and considered much later than when it is medically optimal. By the time surgery is chosen, the person has developed more advanced disease states and possibly gained more weight. Surgery performed earlier could have paused and reversed the disease processes that placed this person in the situation.

Develop and incorporate the lifestyle you will need to adopt after weight loss surgery before any procedure. This helps increase the likelihood of both a successful surgery and long term continued successful weight management.

## 10.1. Pre-Surgery

Not everyone is a good candidate for bariatric surgery. Surgery is best for those who are able and willing to adhere to post-surgery care. Current indications for bariatric surgery are for those with a BMI over 40 $m/Kg^2$, those with a BMI over 35 $m/Kg^2$ and at least 1 severe comorbidity related to their weight, or for those with a BMI over 30 $m/Kg^2$ who have diabetes or metabolic syndrome.[75]

People with cardiopulmonary disease who carry a high surgery risk should avoid surgery. Those with drug or alcohol abuse problems should not have bariatric surgery, nor should those with uncontrolled severe psychiatric illnesses.[75]

It is critical for the success of any of these surgeries that you understand the risks, benefits, expected outcomes, and alternatives to your surgery. You must also comprehend the required lifestyle changes.[75]

114

Should there be a reversible endocrine or other disorder that causes extra weight, that condition should be addressed and corrected before any surgery proceeds.[75]

Mental illnesses are common in bariatric surgery candidates. As many as 23% of those undergoing weight loss surgery report a current mood disorder with depression being most common.[76] For this reason, a psychiatric evaluation is recommended.

Before surgery, there are several evaluations to expect:

- All age and risk-appropriate cancer screenings will be performed.
- A complete review of your medical history and physical exam by your doctor.
- A laboratory evaluation.
- A nutritional evaluation. Many payors (insurance companies) require at least 6 months of non-surgical weight loss interventions before surgery.
- A cardiopulmonary evaluation which potentially might include a sleep study, electrocardiogram, echocardiogram, or other tests.
- A psycho-social and behavioral evaluation.
- A gastroenterology evaluation.
- Counseling to stop using tobacco.
- Counseling regarding pregnancy. It is not recommended to become pregnant for 12 to 18 months after surgery.

## 10.2. Surgical Procedures

There are three common types of bariatric surgeries we will discuss here. These procedures are the laparoscopic adjustable gastric banding, laparoscopic sleeve gastrectomy, and Roux-en-Y gastric bypass.[75]

## 10.2.1. Laparoscopic Adjustable Gastric Banding

The laparoscopic adjustable gastric banding procedure places an adjustable, hollow band made out of silicone around the upper stomach. Once inflated, this band reduces the capacity of the stomach, resulting in early satiety. The band around the stomach is inflated through a port inserted just under the skin. This allows for the band to be inflated (increasing the restrictive effects) or deflated (allowing for less restriction).

With the gastric banding procedure, people typically lose around 44% of their excess body weight. Potential complications include band erosion or slipping. Should that happen, the band becomes ineffective. There is always a risk for the need of a potential revision or removal of the device. Sometimes a leak in the reservoir occurs and the band cannot be inflated.[75]

The band procedure caries higher rates of complications compared with the other two common bariatric surgeries. The other bariatric procedures are also more effective for weight loss. For these reasons, the laparoscopic adjustable gastric banding procedure has generally fallen out of favor and is currently the least common bariatric surgery.[75]

## 10.2.2. Sleeve Gastrectomy

The sleeve gastrectomy is a surgical procedure where most of the body of the stomach and all of the fundus is removed. This results in a smaller and tubular-shaped stomach.

People who undergo this surgery can expect to lose 56% of their excess weight. Potential complications include leaking from where the stomach is sutured as well as vomiting.

The mechanism for weight loss in this surgery is a combination of restrictive and hormonal changes. The stomach is reduced to 25% of its previous size. This results in early satiety similar to the gastric banding procedure.

Ghrelin, the hunger hormone, is produced and secreted from the fundus of the stomach. When this part of the stomach is removed, ghrelin levels significantly drop. People feel less hungry and gain more control over their food cravings.

This is an excellent bariatric surgical option and is increasing in popularity. It is the most common bariatric surgical procedure. [75]

## 10.2.3. Roux-en-Y Gastric Bypass

The Roux-en-Y gastric bypass is a more complex surgical procedure. In this surgery, the stomach is bisected to form a small gastric pouch. This pouch is then connected to the second part of the small intestine (jejunum) forming a roux, as food bypasses much of the stomach and the first part of the small intestine (duodenum). The remainder of the stomach, along with the first part of the small intestine (duodenum) are then reattached further down on the small intestine.

These significant anatomical changes result in weight loss through a combination of restrictive and malabsorptive mechanisms. The gastric pouch, whose size is less than 50 ml, provides significant restriction resulting in weight loss. The duodenum, which is normally responsible for much of the enzymatic breakdown of food and absorption of nutrients in the small intestine, is bypassed by all the food and nutrients. Because of this bypass, calories and nutrients are not absorbed as effectively, which results in weight loss from malabsorption.

The gastric bypass is associated with several severe complications. There can be a leak anywhere a lumen was cut and sutured back together. In this surgery, there are many possible locations for this to occur, from the bisection of the stomach to reattaching the duodenum to the jejunum.

With any surgery involving the gastrointestinal tract, a person could experience narrowing of the lumen or even obstruction causing severe distress. They might instead experience dilation of their gastric pouch which reduces the effectiveness of the restrictive action.

Another complication is delayed gastric emptying. Here, food moves through the gastrointestinal system slower than the normal rate. Alternatively, another complication is called Dumping Syndrome which happens within half an hour after a sudden addition of too much food (especially food with sugar) for the small stomach pouch. The food moves quickly into the intestine, which expands rapidly, pulling water out of the body into the intestine to dilute the sugar. This is followed by intestinal distention, crampy abdominal pain, and then diarrhea. Dumping syndrome is avoided by consuming higher protein content and avoiding simple carbohydrates.

Nutritional deficiencies are common complications following this surgical procedure due to the resulting malabsorption. To prevent these deficiencies, people take multiple supplements after their procedure.

The roux-en-Y gastric bypass is a very effective surgery and people can expect to lose 67% of their excess body weight. The five year average total body weight loss for this procedure is 25.5%, whereas for the sleeve gastrectomy, the average weight loss is 18.8%, and for the banding procedure 11.7%.[77] In 2013, the roux-en-Y was the bariatric choice 34.2% of the time.[75] This surgery is a good choice for those who need to lose more weight.

## 10.3. Post-op

Bariatric surgery changes a person's anatomy. This new anatomy forces lifestyle adjustments. It also increases many health risks such as nutritional deficiencies or post-surgical complications.

## 10.3.1. General Management Following Surgery

In general, medications managing comorbidities must be adjusted as you lose weight after surgery. This weight loss can happen rapidly, so both you and your doctor must be on top of this. Diabetes medications need to be decreased to avoid hypoglycemia. Blood pressure medications need to be decreased to avoid hypotension.

Non-steroid anti-inflammatory (NSAIDs) medications can increase the rates of gastric ulcers, erosions, and bleeding. After these types of surgeries, avoid using NSAIDs as they have a higher risk for these events at the locations where the GI tract was reconnected.

Avoid pregnancy for 12 to 18 months following bariatric surgery. You want your weight to stabilize before any pregnancy. Before undergoing a bariatric procedure, develop a contraceptive plan for this period of time.

There are many doctor visits in the first couple of years after bariatric surgery as your doctor follows labs, tests, and checks on how well you tolerate the dietary, behavioral, and physical activity recommendations.

Another concern is bone density changes. Doctors monitor bone density with dual x-ray absorptiometry (DEXA) scans every 2 years. This will demonstrate how dense your supporting skeleton bones are and if anything is needed to be done to prevent bone loss.

Laboratory tests following bariatric surgery are extensive. They include all of the following:

- Complete Blood Count to evaluate for anemia or infection.
- Complete Metabolic Panel to evaluate kidney function, blood sugar, and the liver.
- Lipid Panel to evaluate cholesterol levels and cardiovascular risk.
- Thyroid Stimulating Hormone to evaluate thyroid function.
- Parathyroid Hormone to evaluate parathyroid and calcium function.
- Iron and Folate to evaluate iron deficiency.
- Cobalamin (Vitamin B12) to evaluate for a vitamin B12 deficiency.
- Thiamine (Vitamin B1)level to evaluate for a vitamin B1 deficiency.
- Vitamin D to evaluate for a vitamin D deficiency.
- Phosphate to evaluate for a phosphate deficiency.
- Magnesium to evaluate for a magnesium deficiency.

The roux-en-Y is most strongly associated with the deficiencies these lab tests evaluate. Following a gastric sleeve or gastric banding procedure usually requires less testing.

## 10.3.2. Typical Supplementation After Bariatric Surgery

Following bariatric surgery, it is recommended to consume over 60 g of protein daily. This prevents muscle loss, especially during the initial stages of weight loss.

There are recommended supplementation guides for each bariatric procedure. It is recommended to take 1,200 mg to 2,000 mg of Calcium citrate daily depending on the procedure. This prevents calcium deficiency. People should be concurrently monitored for osteoporosis using DEXA scan testing as well.[75]

Elemental iron is another recommended supplement and should be taken at least two hours apart from the time the calcium supplement is taken. Expected dose for elemental iron supplementation following bariatric surgery is 45 mg to 60 mg per day.[75]

Following surgery, people are expected to take one to two multivitamins a day (depending on which procedure they underwent) in addition to their other supplements. These multivitamins should include iron, thiamine, folic acid, and copper.[75] The folic acid should total at least 400 mg.

Vitamin B12 should be taken daily at 1,000 mcg. It can be taken either as an injection, under the tongue (sublingual), or oral. The vitamin B12 level should be monitored to assure sufficient levels.[75]

Vitamin D helps with calcium absorption and bone homeostasis. The recommended supplementation after bariatric surgery for vitamin D is at least 2,000 IU per day. The desired vitamin D level is over 30 ng/ml and dosing will need to be adjusted to meet that.

## 10.3.3. Nutritional Deficiencies After Bariatric Surgery

Nutritional deficiencies are one of the largest concerns following bariatric surgery. There are 10 deficiencies that we discuss here.

Protein deficiency occurs in 3% to 18% of those following bariatric surgery. It is evidenced by decreased muscle mass, weakness, and sometimes swelling. This deficiency can be evaluated with an albumin level of less than 3.5 mg/dl. This level should be measured every six to 12 months. To prevent protein deficiency, people should consume 60 g to 120 g of protein a day or 1.1 g/Kg of ideal body weight.

Calcium is another common nutritional deficiency with a prevalence of 10%. Its symptoms include muscle spasms, skin sensations (paraesthesias), and osteopenia or osteoporosis. Ionized calcium is measured and considered deficient if less than 4.48 mg/dl. Calcium is screened for, along with parathyroid hormone, every six to 12 months. Supplementation with calcium and vitamin D can help prevent this deficiency.[78]

Thiamine deficiency occurs frequently following the roux-en-Y procedure with rates as high as 49%. It is initially screened for every three to six months with a serum thiamine level. This level should be above 10 mcg/L. This deficiency can result in problems with the peripheral nervous system as difficulties walking, poor reflexes, pain, vomiting, numbness and more. It also affects the cardiovascular system with increased heart rate and swelling in the arms and legs. There can also be emotional and mental disturbances. It is prevented with a supplement of 6 mg per day, usually in a multivitamin.[78]

A deficiency of vitamin B12, or cobalamin, results in anemia, fatigue, sensory deficits, and even dementia.

Screening is performed by measuring vitamin B12 and drawn every six to 12 months. Supplementation can help prevent this deficiency.[78]

Folic acid is deficient with a folate level of less than 4 nmol/L. Folic acid deficiency also results in anemia and fatigue. If it occurs during pregnancy, it can affect the baby's development. It should be measured every six to 12 months and can be supplemented with 1,000 mcg daily to prevent a deficiency.[78]

Vitamin D deficiency is found in those with a level less than 20 ng/ml. It is a common deficiency, being found in 25% to 80% of those following bariatric surgery. It results in fractures, depression, muscle aches, and bone pain. Screening is done every six to 12 months. Supplementation with 1,200 IU to 2,000 IU daily can prevent the deficiency.[78]

Symptoms of iron deficiency are anemia, fatigue, cracking and inflammation in the corners of the mouth, tongue soreness, and difficulty breathing with exertion. Iron levels should be above 40 mcg/dl and the iron saturation level above 15%. Screening for iron deficiency, after surgery, is performed every six to 12 months. Supplementation can prevent iron deficiency.[78]

Zinc deficiency is measured with a plasma zinc level and confirmed with a level of less than 11 mcmol/L. Low zinc levels lead to poor wound healing, skin lesions, and hair loss. It can be screened annually. There is no supplement recommendation to prevent a deficiency, though if found to be low, it can be supplemented to bring the level back to normal.[78]

Vitamin A is only optionally screened for. A deficiency results in dry hair, poor immunity, and dry eyes. It occurs in up to 12.5% of those who underwent the Roux-en-Y procedure. Vitamin A deficiency can be prevented with supplementation.[78]

Copper deficiency is rare, occurring in only 2% of those who had Roux-en-Y surgery. Symptoms include a spastic gait, peripheral neuropathy, skin sensations, low blood cell counts, fatigue, and more. There are no recommendations for screening but if on zinc, it can be monitored. Normal levels are above 11 mcmol/L. Prevention supplementation levels are 2 mg per day.[78]

## 10.3.4. Summary

Bariatric surgery is an appropriate choice for many people with extra weight. It is a way to help people succeed and live a healthier life. Following surgery, the perception of quality of life improves, as do medical conditions such as cholesterol, diabetes, and blood pressure.[75]

Weight loss surgery significantly improves mortality from disease, including cardiovascular disease and cancer. There is a significant reduction in 10-year all-cause mortality among those who undergo weight loss surgery.[75]

Of these surgical options, the Roux-en-Y procedure results in the most weight loss, followed by the gastric sleeve, and then the gastric banding procedure.[75] Given the complication rates of the gastric banding and the relative lack of weight loss compared with the other procedures, gastric banding is decreasing in popularity as a weight loss surgical choice.

A concern always exists for weight regain following bariatric surgery. Reviewing the causes of weight regain in those who have had a weight loss surgical procedure, one study found five main reasons. These reasons were nutritional indiscretions, mental health issues, endocrine and metabolic alterations, physical inactivity, and anatomic surgical failures.[75]

Nutritional indiscretions and physical inactivity are potentially avoidable with education and support. Understanding expectations before undergoing surgery and preparing for the post-surgical lifestyle, while adopting some good habits before surgery would help. Mental health issues along with endocrine and metabolic alterations can be managed with close physician supervision to minimize weight regain. Work to develop a personal relationship with your primary care physician. Anatomic surgical failure is outside of the patient's control but can be recognized and addressed early by the surgeon to prevent excessive weight regain.

## *10.4. Body Contouring Surgery*

With weight loss, fat cells shrink in size, but the enlarged skin size remains. With significant weight loss, excess skin can cause significant functional impairment. Body contouring surgery (BCS) might be a desired option.

Consider body contouring surgery after weight stability is achieved for over one year. Candidates for this surgery are over the age of 16, do not smoke, and have good social support.[76]

The most common complications of BCS are infection and wound dehiscence (wound re-opening).[76] People undergoing BCS often experience poor wound healing, which would be exacerbated by smoking. Good social support helps improve long term rates of surgical success.

Overall, BCS can be a positive experience and improve a person's physical and mental well-being. It might also protect against weight regain.[76]

# 11. Final Thoughts

*"All great achievements require time."*

*~Maya Angelou~*

In the modern world, where calorie-dense food is plentiful, food marketing effective, and highly processed foods easy to come by, maintaining normal weight requires active management. Your weight does not reflect your self-control or self-motivation. Weight is a product of a complex mix of genetics, environment, hormones, sleep, dietary choices, stress, activity level, medical conditions, medications, and more.

Some personal responsibility accounts for a person's weight. This responsibility, though, is most often not as significant a factor as commonly thought. There are many aspects of weight outside of a person's control; whether their mother smoked during pregnancy, they were born premature, they were breastfed, how many antibiotics they were exposed to as a child, if they gained extra weight as a child or adolescent, their genetics, and so on.

Overall, obesity is an endocrine disease. Many hormones perform the complex dance within the body that results in weight homeostasis. Hormones and signaling proteins which were discussed throughout this book include

127

insulin, leptin, ghrelin, adiponectin, CCK, GLP-1, cortisol, norepinephrine, dopamine, serotonin, GABA, CART, NPY, POMC, estrogen, progesterone, and testosterone. Adjusting your life to optimize how these hormones interact with each other and function to take advantage of how they work is how you gain long term success with your weight management.

The ideal weight management strategy for each person is an individualized one. Everyone has their particular strengths, weaknesses, goals, and challenges. Most concisely, weight management is reduced to diet, sleep, stress control, social support, physical activity, medication management, and bariatric surgery.

- At the core of successful weight management are healthy dietary choices, portion control, and some level of calorie restriction.

- Ideal sleep is restful and restorative lasting between seven and nine hours a night.

- Stress should be managed purposely by directly addressing the causes of stress and utilizing general techniques to reduce stress.

- Weight management success improves with social support. Work together with friends and family, share the weight loss journey, hold each other accountable, share good habits to reinforce the successes between all.

- Physical activity is a critical key to weight maintenance following weight loss. Activity goals are 150 to 300 minutes of moderate level activity every week (30 minutes to 60 minutes daily). Combined with continued calorie restriction, this will help prevent weight regain.

- Medical conditions should be preferentially treated with medications that are weight losing or weight neutral to avoid unnecessary weight gain.
- Weight loss medications are available that affect receptors in the brain and gastrointestinal tract to encourage earlier satiety, increased sensation of fullness, and reduction in appetite.
- Bariatric surgery is an option that should be contemplated early in the weight loss journey. Weight loss surgery is associated with improvements in all-cause mortality. Weight loss is significant and disease processes, such as diabetes, are dramatically affected.

You now have the knowledge and the tools to gain control of your weight. You have strategies you can employ. You have techniques you can act on. Develop your weight management team consisting of your family, friends, doctor, dietitian, therapist, physical trainer, and more. Your journey began with the first page of this book and will continue long after you turn the last page. Your life journey is the fun part!

Matthew Rensberry, MD, MBA

# 12. Appendices

# *Appendix 1: Weight-Related Calculations*

Here is a collection of calculations mentioned throughout the book. You can perform these calculations easily at this website: matthew.rensberry.com.

- Calculate your **body mass index (BMI)**
    - (Weight in Kg)/(Height in m)$^2$
- Calculate **clinically meaningful weight loss** (5% to 10%)
    - For clinically meaningful weight loss, you need to lose between this amount (e.g.: If you weigh 260 lbs):
        - (Your Weight) (0.05) = (260) (0.05) = 13 lbs
        - (Your Weight) (0.1) = (260) (0.1) = 26 lbs
- Estimate your **daily caloric goal** for weight loss
    - This is the number of calories to aim for daily.
        - Males = 66.5 + 13.75 (weight in Kg) + 5.003 (height in cm) – 6.755 (age) - 500

- - Females = 655.1 + 9.563 (weight in Kg) + 1.850 (height in cm) – 4.676 (age) - 500
- Calculate your **estimated percent body fat**
  - Estimated Percent Body fat = 1.2 (BMI) + 0.23 (age) – 10.8 (gender) - 5.4
  - Where gender = '1' for men and '0' for women
- Calculate the amount of **calories from added sugar**
  - Current recommendations for added sugar is less than 100 calories for women and less than 150 calories for men. (e.g.: 12 oz Coca-Cola with 39 g added sugars)
  - (grams of added sugar)*4 = (39)*4 = 156 calories
- Calculate your **sleep efficiency** for sleep restriction therapy
  - Time in bed (TIB) is the total amount of time trying to sleep or sleeping (e.g.: 9 hours)
  - Total Sleep Time (TST) is the total amount of time sleeping (e.g.: 6 hours)
  - (TST/TIB) 100 = (6/9)*100 = 0.66*100 = 66% sleep efficiency

There is an easy to use calculator online at matthew.rensberry.com for you to easily calculate your BMI, clinically meaningful weight loss goal, daily caloric goal, and estimated percent body fat.

# *Appendix 2: Smartphone Applications*

Smartphones provide a toolbox for easy access to tools to help you on your weight journey. New applications are always appearing. Try out several different types of applications to see which one works best for you.

- **Stress and Anxiety Applications:**
  - <u>Sanvello</u>: Sanvello enables you to track your daily activities, and then identify things that trigger stress and anxiety. After identifying what triggers your stress and anxiety, you can then address them and work to eliminate them. It uses cognitive behavioral therapy to help address stress and anxiety.

  - <u>Rootd</u>: Rootd provides mindfulness exercises and step-by-step guides to techniques like diaphragmatic breathing. It is helpful for anxiety and panic attacks. The app has a personal statistics section to encourage you as it shows how many panic attacks you have overcome and lessons completed. There is also an emergency contact button to easily call someone when in distress.

- Breathe2Relax: Breathe2Relax is an app created by the Department of Defense's Center for Tele-health and Technology to help soldiers learn breathing techniques to relieve stress and anxiety. It helps you learn to perform diaphragmatic breathing and control your breathing.

- Stop, Breathe & Think: Stop, Breathe, and Think is a mindfulness app that begins with you selecting your mood. From this, it will suggest what might work best for you at the moment from modalities such as deep breathing to visualizations. It tracks your moods and progress which helps you understand your stress and anxiety better.

- Headspace: Headspace is a meditation app that uses gamification in its experience. It guides you through a variety of meditations and teaches you the basics.

- Calm: Calm provides guided meditations for all levels. It also has relaxation sounds which can even help put you to sleep.

- Happify: Happify's tagline is "Science-Based Activities and Games for Stress and Anxiety Relief." It has different activities to help you improve your mood and learn to control your happiness.

- **Sleep Applications**

  - Sleep Cycle: Sleep cycle is an app that wakes you up during your lightest sleep stage. When you wake up in the middle of deep sleep, you feel groggy and disoriented. This app avoids that by waking you up outside of that timeframe.

  - Sleep Time: Sleep time is an app that works by you placing it on your bed so it can track your sleep time and cycles. It can help you find trends in your sleep so you can have restful and restorative sleep

- <u>Relax Melodies</u>: Relax melodies has a large library of relaxation sounds. It also provides guided meditations and sleep meditations.

- **Calorie Tracking Applications**

  - <u>MyFitnessPal</u>: MyFitnessPal is a calorie tracker with a massive food database, bar-code scanner, and recipe importer. This makes tracking calories very easy. It also can provide social support in the app.

  - <u>LoseIt!</u>: LoseIt is another calorie tracker with a large food database and bar-code scanning. It has a feature to track food by taking a photo of it.

  - <u>FatSecret</u>: FatSecret harnesses the power of social support in weight management. It is a calorie tracker and weight monitor that enables you to interact with others through a chat feature. There are groups you can join with similar goals. It also has a journal to record notes from your weight journey. This app also has a tool where you can share your food, exercise, and weight data with your doctor.

- **Real-life Social Applications**

  - <u>MeetUp</u>: Find local support groups and activities to participate in. This app helps you find other people with the same struggles, goals, and interests. There are MeetUp groups for weight loss, specific diets (like keto groups), and exercise (like walking, running, or cycling groups).

- **Control Your Social Media Applications**
  - <u>Moment</u>: Moment is a screen time tracker to help you analyze how much time you are using on your phone and what apps consume your attention.

  - <u>Space</u>: Space is an app to help you understand your phone usage habits and allows you to set goals to break free from smartphone addiction.

  - <u>Offtime</u>: Offtime provides a way to track and customize your connectivity so you can free yourself from your phone. It provides insights into your phone use and a way to block calls, texts, and notifications as desired. It also can help you set personal restrictions on apps and the Internet.

  - <u>Forest</u>: Forest is a gamified timer to help you focus on things outside of your smartphone. Plant a seed by putting your phone down and as time goes by, the seed grows into a tree.

Smartphone applications change frequently. Visit matthew.rensberry.com for up to date resources.

# Appendix 3: Low Glycemic Index Food Reference

The Low Glycemic Index Diet works with your current diet plan. To use this diet, continue your current calorie and carbohydrate intake but follow these four steps:

1. Make a list of the carbohydrates in your diet. Write down how often you eat vegetables, fruits, bread, grains, cereals, pasta, rice, juices, beans, soups, baked goods, etc.

2. After making this list, find the Glycemic Index for each food. If you have trouble finding a food's GI, look for the ingredients of the food.

   • If the ingredients are highly processed (refined white flour, sugar, corn syrup) rank the food as a high GI food.

   • If the food has mixed ingredients of some processed and some unprocessed ingredients, rank it as a medium GI food.

   • If almost all the ingredients are unprocessed, rank the food as a low GI food.

3. Try to eliminate all the high GI foods (those with a GI over 70) from your diet. Do what you can to remove some of the medium GI foods (those with a GI between 55 and 70) as well.

4. Using a reference of GI food values, identify low GI foods you can substitute into your everyday diet. Should you have a high GI food in a meal, see if you can offset it by consuming something with a very low GI to bring down the average GI of your entire meal.

On the following page is a list of many common foods and their estimated GI value. This list can also be found at matthew.rensberry.com.

Table 1: **Low Glycemic Index Food Reference**

| Food Category | Food | GI Value |
|---|---|---|
| Fruits | Apple | 38 |
| | Apricots, canned | 64 |
| | Apricots, dried | 30 |
| | Apricots, fresh | 57 |
| | Banana | 52 |
| | Cantaloupe | 65 |
| | Cherries | 22 |
| | Dates | 103 |
| | Figs, dried | 61 |
| | Fruit Cocktail | 55 |
| | Grapefruit | 25 |
| | Grapes | 46 |
| | Kiwi | 58 |
| | Mango | 51 |
| | Navel Orange | 42 |

141

| Food Category | Food | GI Value |
| --- | :---: | :---: |
| | Papaya | 56 |
| | Peach, canned | 38 |
| | Peach, fresh | 42 |
| | Pear, canned | 43 |
| | Pear, fresh | 38 |
| | Pineapple, fresh | 66 |
| | Plum | 39 |
| | Prunes | 29 |
| | Raisins | 56 |
| | Strawberries | 40 |
| | Watermelon | 72 |
| Vegetables | Beets | 64 |
| | Broccoli | 10 |
| | Cabbage | 10 |
| | Carrots | 49 |
| | Corn, fresh | 60 |

| Food Category | Food | GI Value |
| --- | --- | --- |
| | Green peas | 48 |
| | Lettuce | 10 |
| | Mushrooms | 10 |
| | Onions | 10 |
| | Parsnips | 97 |
| | Pumpkin | 75 |
| | Red Peppers | 10 |
| Beans | Baked Beans | 48 |
| | Blackeyed Peas, canned | 42 |
| | Chana Dal | 8 |
| | Chickpeas, canned | 42 |
| | Chickpeas, dried | 28 |
| | Kidney Beans, canned | 52 |
| | Kidney Beans, dried | 28 |
| | Lentils | 29 |

| Food Category | Food | GI Value |
|---|---|---|
| | Lima Beans (frozen) | 32 |
| | Yellow Split Peas | 32 |
| Potatoes | Baked | 85 |
| | Canned | 65 |
| | Instant Mashed | 86 |
| | French Fries | 75 |
| | New | 57 |
| | Red Skinned, boiled | 88 |
| | Sweet Potatoes | 44 |
| | White-skinned mashed | 70 |
| | Yam | 37 |
| Rice | Aborio | 69 |
| | Basmati | 58 |
| | Barley, pearled | 25 |
| | Brown | 55 |
| | Buckwheat | 54 |

| Food Category | Food | GI Value |
|---|---|---|
| | Converted, White | 38 |
| | Cornmeal | 68 |
| | Couscous | 65 |
| | Glutinous (Sticky) | 98 |
| | Instant, White | 87 |
| | Long grain, White | 44 |
| | Short grain, White | 72 |
| | Wild rice | 87 |
| Soups | Black Bean | 64 |
| | Lentil | 44 |
| | Minestrone | 39 |
| | Pea | 66 |
| | Tomato | 38 |
| Pasta | Capellini | 45 |
| | Fettuccini (egg) | 32 |
| | Linguine | 46 |

| Food Category | Food | GI Value |
| --- | --- | --- |
| | Macaroni | 47 |
| | Spaghetti, White | 38 |
| | Spaghetti, Whole Wheat | 37 |
| | Spiral Pasta | 43 |
| | Star Pastina | 38 |
| | Rice Vermicelli | 58 |
| Bread | Bagel | 72 |
| | Bread stuffing | 74 |
| | Croissant | 67 |
| | French Baguette | 95 |
| | Hamburger bun | 61 |
| | Kaiser roll | 73 |
| | Pita, whole wheat | 57 |
| | Pumpernickel | 41 |
| | Sourdough | 53 |

| Food Category | Food | GI Value |
|---|---|---|
| | Stone Ground Whole Wheat | 53 |
| | Taco Shell | 68 |
| | White | 70 |
| | Whole Meal Rye | 58 |
| | Whole Wheat | 77 |
| Bakery | Angel Food Cake | 67 |
| | Blueberry Muffin | 59 |
| | Bran Muffin | 60 |
| | Carrot Muffin | 62 |
| | Doughnut | 76 |
| | Pastry Pie Crust | 59 |
| | Pound Cake | 54 |
| | Scones | 92 |
| | Sponge Cake | 46 |
| Crackers | Graham Crackers | 74 |

| Food Category | Food | GI Value |
|---|---|---|
| | Kavli Crispbread | 71 |
| | Melba Toast | 70 |
| | Rice Cakes | 82 |
| | Rice Crackers | 91 |
| | Ryvita Crispbread | 69 |
| | Soda Crackers | 74 |
| | Stoned Wheat Thins | 67 |
| | Water Crackers | 78 |
| Breakfast Foods | All-Bran with Fiber | 38 |
| | Bran Buds | 47 |
| | Bran Chex | 58 |
| | Bran Flakes | 74 |
| | Cheerios | 74 |
| | Corn Chex | 83 |
| | Corn Flakes | 92 |
| | Cream of Wheat | 66 |

| Food Category | Food | GI Value |
| --- | --- | --- |
| | Cream of Wheat Instant | 74 |
| | Grapenuts | 71 |
| | Muesli | 43 |
| | Oat Bran | 55 |
| | Pancakes | 67 |
| | Puffed Wheat | 67 |
| | Quick Oats (One Minute) | 66 |
| | Raisin Bran | 61 |
| | Rice Krispies | 82 |
| | Shredded Wheat | 75 |
| | Special K | 69 |
| | Waffles | 76 |
| Dairy | Ice cream, low fat | 43 |
| | Ice cream, premium | 38 |
| | Skim milk | 32 |

| Food Category | Food | GI Value |
|---|---|---|
| | Whole milk | 31 |
| | Yogurt, artificially sweetened | 14 |
| | Yogurt, sweetened | 33 |
| Cookies | Butter | 47 |
| | Chocolate Chip | 44 |
| | Fudge | 57 |
| | Oatmeal | 55 |
| | Shortbread | 64 |
| | Vanilla Creme Filled Wafers | 50 |
| Snacks | Cashews | 22 |
| | Corn Chips | 63 |
| | Hummus | 6 |
| | Kudos Bar | 62 |
| | Jelly Beans | 78 |
| | M&M Peanut Candies | 33 |

| Food Category | Food | GI Value |
| --- | :---: | :---: |
| | Milk Chocolate | 43 |
| | Peanuts | 15 |
| | Popcorn | 72 |
| | Potato Chips | 57 |
| | Pretzels | 83 |
| | Walnuts | 15 |
| Juices | Apple | 40 |
| | Cranberry Juice Cocktail | 68 |
| | Grapefruit | 48 |
| | Orange | 53 |
| | Pineapple | 46 |
| | Tomato | 38 |

# Appendix 4: FODMAP Food Reference

A low fermentable oligo-, di-, and monosaccharides and polyols (FODMAP) diet is helpful for those with irritable bowel syndrome and other gastrointestinal distress. To use the diet, you try to eat as few FODMAPs as possible for six to eight weeks. After symptoms have improved, you can gradually reintroduce foods with higher fermentable carbohydrates to determine your tolerance to specific fermentable carbohydrates. Avoid those which trigger symptoms.

On the following page is a list of many common low and high FODMAP foods. This list can also be found at matthew.rensberry.com.

Appendices

## Table 2: **FODMAP Food Reference**

| Category | Low FODMAP Foods | High FODMAP Foods |
|---|---|---|
| Vegetables and Legumes | Bamboo shoots | Garlic |
| | Bean sprouts | Onions |
| | Broccoli | Asparagus |
| | Cabbage | Beans |
| | Carrots | Cauliflower |
| | Celery | Cabbage, savoy |
| | Chickpeas | Mange tout |
| | Corn | Mushrooms |
| | Cucumber | Peas |
| | Eggplant | Scallions / spring onions (white part) |
| | Green beans | |
| | Green pepper | |
| | Kale | |
| | Lettuce | |

| Category | Low FODMAP Foods | High FODMAP Foods |
| --- | --- | --- |
| | Parsnip | |
| | Potato | |
| | Pumpkin | |
| | Red peppers | |
| | Scallions/spring onions (green part) | |
| | Squash | |
| | Sweet potato | |
| | Tomatoes | |
| | Turnip | |
| Fruit | Bananas, unripe | Apples |
| | Blueberries | Apricot |
| | Cranberry | Bananas, ripe |
| | Clementine | Blackberries |
| | Grapes | Grapefruit |
| | Melons | Mango |
| | Kiwifruit | Peaches |

| Category | Low FODMAP Foods | High FODMAP Foods |
|---|---|---|
| | Orange | Plums |
| | Pineapple | Raisins |
| | Raspberry | Watermelon |
| | Rhubarb | |
| | Strawberry | |
| Meats | Beef | Chorizo |
| | Chicken | Sausages |
| | Fresh Fish | Processed meat |
| | Lamb | |
| | Pork | |
| | Quorn mince | |
| | Tuna | |
| Bread, Pasta, Cereals, Grains | Oats | Barley |
| | Quinoa | Bran |
| | Gluten-free foods | Couscous |
| | Buckwheat | Gnocchi |
| | Chips | Granola |

| Category | Low FODMAP Foods | High FODMAP Foods |
|---|---|---|
| | Cornflour | Muesli |
| | Oatmeal | Muffins |
| | Popcorn | Rye |
| | Pretzels | Semolina |
| | Rice | Spelt |
| | Tortilla chips | Wheat foods |
| Nuts and Seeds | Almonds | Cashews |
| | Chestnuts | Pistachio |
| | Hazelnuts | |
| | Macadamia nuts | |
| | Peanuts | |
| | Pecans | |
| | Poppy seeds | |
| | Pumpkin seeds | |
| | Sesame seeds | |
| | Sunflower seeds | |
| | Walnuts | |

| Category | Low FODMAP Foods | High FODMAP Foods |
|---|---|---|
| Dairy, Eggs, Cheese | Almond milk | Cow milk |
| | Coconut milk | Goat milk |
| | Hemp milk | Soy milk |
| | Lactose-free milk | Buttermilk |
| | Oat milk | Cream |
| | Rice milk | Custard |
| | Butter | Greek yogurt |
| | Dark chocolate | Ice cream |
| | Eggs | Sour cream |
| | Milk chocolate | Yogurt |
| | White chocolate | Cream cheese |
| | Brie | Ricotta cheese |
| | Camembert | |
| | Cheddar | |
| | Cottage cheese | |
| | Feta | |
| | Mozzarella | |

| Category | Low FODMAP Foods | High FODMAP Foods |
| --- | --- | --- |
| | Parmesan | |
| | Swiss | |
| Condiments | Barbecue sauce | Hummus dip |
| | Chutney | Mixed berry jam |
| | Garlic infused oil | Cream-based pasta sauce |
| | Golden syrup | Relish |
| | Strawberry jam | Tzatziki dip |
| | Mayonnaise | |
| | Mustard | |
| | Soy sauce | |
| | Tomato sauce | |
| Sweeteners | Aspartame | Agave |
| | Acesulfame K | High Fructose Corn Syrup |
| | Glucose | Honey |
| | Saccharine | Inulin |
| | Stevia | Isomalt |
| | Sucralose | Malttol |

| Category | Low FODMAP Foods | High FODMAP Foods |
|---|---|---|
|  | Sugar | Mannitol |
|  |  | Sorbitol |
|  |  | Xylitol |
| Drinks | Beer | Apple juice |
|  | Black coffee | Coconut water |
|  | Orange juice | Fennel tea |
|  | Peppermint tea | Herbal tea |
|  | Water | Kombucha |
|  | Wine | Mango juice |
|  |  | Pear juice |
|  |  | Rum |
|  |  | Sodas with high fructose corn syrup |

# 13. Index

Adiponectin: 50,61,81,108,127

Anemia: 11,62-63,120,122-123

Anxiety: 8,66-77,79,87,100,104

Antidepressants: 56-57,87,100

Antihistamines: 56-58

Apnea-hypopnea index (AHI): 60

Arrhythmias: 10,58,954

Bacteroidetes: 41,107

Binge eating disorder: 89

Body mass index: 1,3,5,9,45,50,61,99,101,114

CART: 35-36,128

Cholecystokinin (CCK): 28-29,35,128

Continuous positive airway pressure (CPAP): 60-62

Cortisol: 65-67,74,94,128

Dementia: 56,122

Depression: 1,8,49,57,67,75,87,94,103,115,123

Diabetes: 3-4,6,8-9,11,28,30,32-33,36,39,50,60,
    90-93,95,99-101,103,119,124,129

Diaphragmatic breathing: 72

Dopamine: 62-63,75,87-89,102,104,128

Dumping syndrome: 118

Estrogen: 7,95,128

Exercise: 1,6,35,39-40,53,63,71-75,79-83,97,101,
    109

Fatty acid: 22,28,39,61,107

Firmicutes: 41

Fiber: 22-23,32,40,106

Functional gastrointestinal syndrome: 34

Gamma-aminobutyric acid (GABA): 104,128

Gall bladder/gallstones: 8,36

Ghrelin: 31-33,50-51,65,67,117,128

Glaucoma: 58,100,104

Glucagon-like peptide-1/Incretins: 51,91-93,103,128

Glucagon: 38-39

Gluconeogenesis: 39

Glucose: 8,10-12,21-24,32-33,35,38-39,57,90-93,103,
    107,110

Glycogen: 22,38-39

Hypertension: 9,12,36-37,50,65,99,103

Hypothalamus: 22,28,51,88-89,92,94,99,101-104,108

Hypothyroidism: 8,94

Inflammation: 30-31,60-61,65,67,107,123

Insulin: 4,8,11,21-24,30-33,38,40,57,60,65,90-93,106,
    110,128

Inflammatory bowel disease: 34

Intermittent fasting: 40

Ketones: 39

Lean body mass: 80

Leptin: 22,30-31,35,40,50,60-61,80-81,104,108,128

Medroxyprogesterone: 96

Melatonin: 56,58

Metabolic syndrome: 12,114

Microbiome: 26,40-41,47,77

Neuropathy: 62,124

Non-alcoholic fatty liver: 7,11

Norepinephrine: 87-89,99,102,104,128

Neuropeptide Y (NPY): 35,65-67,128

Obstructive sleep apnea: 4,7,59,99

Overactive bladder: 59

Pancreas: 21,28,91

Proopiomelanocortin (POMC): 102,128

Portion size: 20,30,42-43,44-46,82

Progressive muscle relaxation: 72

Progesterone: 95-96,128

Reflux (acid reflux): 7,60

Relaxation techniques: 69,71-72

Restless leg syndrome: 59,62

Satiety: 28-32,46,51,61,88-89,92,101-102,104,106,
108-109,111,116-117,129

Serotonin: 30,57-58,65-67,87,101-102,11,128

Sleep: 4,6-7,32,40,49-63,72,75,79,99,115,127-128

Sleep hygiene: 52

Sleep restriction therapy: 54,56

SMART goals: 13-15

Small intestinal bacterial overgrowth (SIBO): 34

Smoking: 53,78,87,103,125

Stress: 6,32,65-72,74-77,79,94,118,127-128

Stroke: 8,50

Thyroid: 93-94,103,120

Testosterone: 7,11,128

Triglyceride: 4,12,22,39,109

Vitamin B12 (Cyanocobalamin): 10,11,110-111, 120-123

Vitamin D: 10-11,110,120-123

# About the Author

Matthew Rensberry, MD grew up in Central America where he participated with several medical mission teams and developed a love for medicine. He attended Olivet Nazarene University and then studied medicine at The Ohio State University College of Medicine. While there, Matthew joined the United States Army. After medical school, he joined the residency at Fort Hood in Texas. Following residency, he was assigned to the 1st Brigade in the 1st Cavalry Division as their Brigade Surgeon. He deployed for a year to Iraq and Kuwait.

Following his time in the US Army, Dr. Rensberry moved to central Florida and became a faculty member and the medical director for the AdventHealth Family Medicine Program. In 2018, he resigned that position to open a private direct primary care practice.

Matthew is married to Erica, has two children, and three dogs. He enjoys jogging, cycling, hiking, stand-up-paddleboarding, and many other excuses to spend time outdoors.

Dr. Rensberry would love to hear from you! E-mail your thoughts, comments, and questions to: dr.rensberry@anchor-dpc.com. Visit his website at matthew.rensberry.com or his clinic's website at anchor-dpc.com.

# Footnotes

1  Ogden CL, Lamb MM, Carroll MD, Flegal KM. Obesity and socioeconomic status in adults: United States, 2005-2008. *NCHS Data Brief*. 2010;(50):1-8.

2  Finkelstein EA, Trogdon JG, Cohen JW, Dietz W. Annual medical spending attributable to obesity: Payer-and service-specific estimates. *Health Aff (Millwood)*. 2009;28(5):w822-831. doi:10.1377/hlthaff.28.5.w822

3  Ogden CL, Lamb MM, Carroll MD, Flegal KM. Obesity and socioeconomic status in adults: United States, 2005-2008. *NCHS Data Brief*. 2010;(50):1-8.

4  Fortenberry K, Ricks J, Kovach FE. Clinical inquiry. How much does weight loss affect hypertension? *J Fam Pract*. 2013;62(5):258-259.

5  Notara V, Magriplis E, Prapas C, et al. Parental weight status and early adolescence body weight in association with socioeconomic factors. *J Educ Health Promot*. 2019;8:77. doi:10.4103/jehp.jehp_14_19

6  Rito AI, Buoncristiano M, Spinelli A, et al. Association between Characteristics at Birth, Breastfeeding and Obesity in 22 Countries: The WHO European Childhood Obesity Surveillance InitiativeCOSI 2015/2017. *Obes Facts*. 2019;12(2):226-243. doi:10.1159/000500425

7  Nammi S, Koka S, Chinnala KM, Boini KM. Obesity: An overview on its current perspectives and treatment options. *Nutrition Journal*. 2004;3(1):3. doi:10.1186/1475-2891-3-3

8  Clinical guidelines on the identification, evaluation, and treatment of overweight and obesity in adults: Executive summary. Expert Panel on the Identification, Evaluation, and Treatment of Overweight in Adults. *The American Journal of Clinical Nutrition*. 1998;68(4):899-917. doi:10.1093/ajcn/68.4.899

9  Weight Calculations. Matthew Rensberry. https://matthew.rensberry.com/weight-calculator/.

10 Redman LM, Smith SR, Burton JH, Martin CK, Il'yasova D, Ravussin E. Metabolic Slowing and Reduced Oxidative Damage with Sustained Caloric Restriction Support the Rate of Living and Oxidative Damage Theories of Aging. *Cell Metabolism*. 2018;27(4):805-815.e4. doi:10.1016/j.cmet.2018.02.019

11 Johnson RK, Appel LJ, Brands M, et al. Dietary sugars intake and cardiovascular health: A scientific statement from the

American Heart Association. *Circulation*. 2009;120(11):1011-1020. doi:10.1161/CIRCULATIONAHA.109.192627

12 American Heart Association. Added Sugars. Added Sugars. https://www.heart.org/en/healthy-living/healthy-eating/eat-smart/sugar/added-sugars. Published April 17, 2018.

13 Malik VS, Hu FB. Fructose and Cardiometabolic Health: What the Evidence From Sugar-Sweetened Beverages Tells Us. *J Am Coll Cardiol*. 2015;66(14):1615-1624. doi:10.1016/j.jacc.2015.08.025

14 Pan A, Hu FB. Effects of carbohydrates on satiety: Differences between liquid and solid food. *Curr Opin Clin Nutr Metab Care*. 2011;14(4):385-390. doi:10.1097/MCO.0b013e328346df36

15 Collin LJ, Judd S, Safford M, Vaccarino V, Welsh JA. Association of Sugary Beverage Consumption With Mortality Risk in US Adults: A Secondary Analysis of Data From the REGARDS Study. *JAMA Netw Open*. 2019;2(5):e193121. doi:10.1001/jamanetworkopen.2019.3121

16 Harpaz D, Yeo LP, Cecchini F, et al. Measuring Artificial Sweeteners Toxicity Using a Bioluminescent Bacterial Panel. *Molecules*. 2018;23(10). 10.3390/molecules23102454

17 Ebbeling CB, Feldman HA, Klein GL, et al. Effects of a low carbohydrate diet on energy expenditure during weight loss maintenance: Randomized trial. *BMJ*. 2018;363:k4583. 10.1136/bmj.k4583

18 La Berge AF. How the Ideology of Low Fat Conquered America. *Journal of the History of Medicine and Allied Sciences*. 2008;63(2):139-177. 10.1093/jhmas/jrn001

19 Aeberli I, Gerber PA, Hochuli M, et al. Low to moderate sugar-sweetened beverage consumption impairs glucose and lipid metabolism and promotes inflammation in healthy young men: A randomized controlled trial. *Am J Clin Nutr*. 2011;94(2):479-485. 10.3945/ajcn.111.013540

20 Lopez-Alarcon M, Perichart-Perera O, Flores-Huerta S, et al. Excessive refined carbohydrates and scarce micronutrients intakes increase inflammatory mediators and insulin resistance in prepubertal and pubertal obese children independently of obesity. *Mediators Inflamm*. 2014;2014:849031. 10.1155/2014/849031

21 Spadaro PA, Naug HL, DU Toit EF, Donner D, Colson NJ. A refined high carbohydrate diet is associated with changes in

the serotonin pathway and visceral obesity. *Genet Res (Camb)*. 2015;97:e23. 10.1017/S0016672315000233

22 Orlich MJ, Singh PN, Sabate J, et al. Vegetarian dietary patterns and mortality in Adventist Health Study 2. *JAMA Intern Med*. 2013;173(13):1230-1238. 10.1001/jamainternmed.2013.6473

23 Rizzo NS, Jaceldo-Siegl K, Sabate J, Fraser GE. Nutrient profiles of vegetarian and nonvegetarian dietary patterns. *J Acad Nutr Diet*. 2013;113(12):1610-1619. 10.1016/j.jand.2013.06.349

24 Tonstad S, Stewart K, Oda K, Batech M, Herring RP, Fraser GE. Vegetarian diets and incidence of diabetes in the Adventist Health Study-2. *Nutr Metab Cardiovasc Dis*. 2013;23(4):292-299. 10.1016/j.numecd.2011.07.004

25 Goff LM, Cowland DE, Hooper L, Frost GS. Low glycaemic index diets and blood lipids: A systematic review and meta-analysis of randomised controlled trials. *Nutr Metab Cardiovasc Dis*. 2013;23(1):1-10. 10.1016/j.numecd.2012.06.002

26 Larsen TM, Dalskov S-M, van Baak M, et al. Diets with high or low protein content and glycemic index for weight-loss maintenance. *N Engl J Med*. 2010;363(22):2102-2113. 10.1056/NEJMoa1007137

27 Barrett JS. Extending our knowledge of fermentable, short-chain carbohydrates for managing gastrointestinal symptoms. *Nutr Clin Pract*. 2013;28(3):300-306. 10.1177/0884533613485790

28 Dandekar MP, Singru PS, Kokare DM, Subhedar NK. Cocaine- and amphetamine-regulated transcript peptide plays a role in the manifestation of depression: Social isolation and olfactory bulbectomy models reveal unifying principles. *Neuropsychopharmacology*. 2009;34(5):1288-1300. 10.1038/npp.2008.201

29 Mediterranean Diet. Veterans Association; 2015. https://www.nutrition.va.gov/docs/UpdatedPatientEd/Mediter raneandiet.pdf. Accessed July 10, 2018.

30 *IN BRIEF: Your Guide To Lowering Your Blood Pressure With DASH*. National Heart, Lung, and Blood Institute; 2015. https://www.nhlbi.nih.gov/files/docs/public/heart/dash_brief.p df. Accessed July 5, 2018.

170

31 *YOUR GUIDE TO Lowering Your Blood Pressure With DASH*. National Heart, Lung, and Blood Institute, National Institutes of Health; 2006. https://www.nhlbi.nih.gov/files/docs/public/heart/new_dash.pdf. Accessed July 5, 2018.

32 Gardner CD, Trepanowski JF, Del Gobbo LC, et al. Effect of Low-Fat vs Low-Carbohydrate Diet on 12-Month Weight Loss in Overweight Adults and the Association With Genotype Pattern or Insulin Secretion: The DIETFITS Randomized Clinical Trial. *JAMA*. 2018;319(7):667-679. 10.1001/jama.2018.0245

33 Halberg N, Henriksen M, Soderhamn N, et al. Effect of intermittent fasting and refeeding on insulin action in healthy men. *J Appl Physiol (1985)*. 2005;99(6):2128-2136. 10.1152/japplphysiol.00683.2005

34 Semova I, Carten JD, Stombaugh J, et al. Microbiota regulate intestinal absorption and metabolism of fatty acids in the zebrafish. *Cell Host Microbe*. 2012;12(3):277-288. 10.1016/j.chom.2012.08.003

35 Ley RE, Backhed F, Turnbaugh P, Lozupone CA, Knight RD, Gordon JI. Obesity alters gut microbial ecology. *Proc Natl Acad Sci U S A*. 2005;102(31):11070-11075. 10.1073/pnas.0504978102

36 Ley RE, Turnbaugh PJ, Klein S, Gordon JI. Microbial ecology: Human gut microbes associated with obesity. *Nature*. 2006;444(7122):1022-1023. 10.1038/4441022a

37 Piernas C, Popkin BM. Food portion patterns and trends among U.S. children and the relationship to total eating occasion size, 1977-2006. *J Nutr*. 2011;141(6):1159-1164. 10.3945/jn.111.138727

38 Division of Nutrition and Physical Activity. *Research to Practice Series No. 2: Portion Size*. Atlanta: Centers for Disease Control and Prevention; 2006. https://www.cdc.gov/nccdphp/dnpa/nutrition/pdf/portion_size_research.pdf.

39 James Clear. *Atomic Habits: An Easy & Proven Way to Build Good Habits & Break Bad Ones*. Avery; 2018.

40 Centers for Disease Control and Prevention. Short Sleep Duration Among US Adults. CDC - Data and Statistics. https://www.cdc.gov/sleep/data_statistics.html. Published May 2, 2017. Accessed April 16, 2019.

41 Watson NF, Badr MS, Belenky G, et al. Recommended Amount of Sleep for a Healthy Adult: A Joint Consensus Statement of the American Academy of Sleep Medicine and Sleep Research Society. *J Clin Sleep Med*. 2015;11(6):591-592. 10.5664/jcsm.4758

42 Reutrakul S, Van Cauter E. Sleep influences on obesity, insulin resistance, and risk of type 2 diabetes. *Metabolism*. 2018;84:56-66. 10.1016/j.metabol.2018.02.010

43 Sorscher AJ. Insomnia: Getting to the cause, facilitating relief. *J Fam Pract*. 2017;66(4):216-225.

44 Neubauer DN. A review of ramelteon in the treatment of sleep disorders. *Neuropsychiatr Dis Treat*. 2008;4(1):69-79. 10.2147/ndt.s483

45 Romero-Corral A, Caples SM, Lopez-Jimenez F, Somers VK. Interactions between obesity and obstructive sleep apnea: Implications for treatment. *Chest*. 2010;137(3):711-719. 10.1378/chest.09-0360

46 Restless Legs Syndrome Fact Sheet. National Institute of Neurological Disorders and Stroke. https://www.ninds.nih.gov/Disorders/Patient-Caregiver-Education/Fact-Sheets/Restless-Legs-Syndrome-Fact-Sheet. Published May 14, 2019. Accessed June 5, 2019.

47 Gao X, Schwarzschild MA, Wang H, Ascherio A. Obesity and restless legs syndrome in men and women. *Neurology*. 2009;72(14):1255-1261. 10.1212/01.wnl.0000345673.35676.1c

48 Bose M, Olivan B, Laferrere B. Stress and obesity: The role of the hypothalamic-pituitary-adrenal axis in metabolic disease. *Curr Opin Endocrinol Diabetes Obes*. 2009;16(5):340-346. 10.1097/MED.0b013e32832fa137

49 Wurtman RJ, Wurtman JJ. Brain serotonin, carbohydrate-craving, obesity and depression. *Obes Res*. 1995;3 Suppl 4:477S-480S.

50 Chuang J-C, Zigman JM. Ghrelin's Roles in Stress, Mood, and Anxiety Regulation. *Int J Pept*. 2010;2010. doi:10.1155/2010/460549

51 Lee LO, James P, Zevon ES, et al. Optimism is associated with exceptional longevity in 2 epidemiologic cohorts of men and women. *Proc Natl Acad Sci U S A*. August 2019. doi:10.1073/pnas.1900712116

52 Vannucci A, Flannery KM, Ohannessian CM. Social media use and anxiety in emerging adults. *J Affect Disord*. 2017;207:163-166. 10.1016/j.jad.2016.08.040

53 Hoge E, Bickham D, Cantor J. Digital Media, Anxiety, and Depression in Children. *Pediatrics*. 2017;140(Suppl 2):S76-S80. 10.1542/peds.2016-1758G

54 Christakis NA, Fowler JH. The spread of obesity in a large social network over 32 years. *N Engl J Med*. 2007;357(4):370-379. 10.1056/NEJMsa066082

55 Becic T, Studenik C, Hoffmann G. Exercise Increases Adiponectin and Reduces Leptin Levels in Prediabetic and Diabetic Individuals: Systematic Review and Meta-Analysis of Randomized Controlled Trials. *Med Sci (Basel)*. 2018;6(4). 10.3390/medsci6040097

56 Piercy KL, Troiano RP, Ballard RM, et al. The Physical Activity Guidelines for Americans. *JAMA*. 2018;320(19):2020-2028. 10.1001/jama.2018.14854

57 Arterburn D, Sofer T, Boudreau MD, et al. Long-Term Weight Change after Initiating Second-Generation Antidepressants. *Journal of Clinical Medicine*. 2016;5(4). 10.3390/jcm5040048

58 Allison KC, Tarves EP. Treatment of night eating syndrome. *The Psychiatric clinics of North America*. 2011;34(4):785-796. 10.1016/j.psc.2011.08.002

59 Campbell JM, Bellman SM, Stephenson MD, Lisy K. Metformin reduces all-cause mortality and diseases of ageing independent of its effect on diabetes control: A systematic review and meta-analysis. *Ageing Res Rev*. 2017;40:31-44. 10.1016/j.arr.2017.08.003

60 9. Pharmacologic Approaches to Glycemic Treatment: Standards of Medical Care in Diabetes—2019. *Diabetes Care*. 2019;42(Supplement 1):S90. 10.2337/dc19-S009

61 Ferrannini G, Hach T, Crowe S, Sanghvi A, Hall KD, Ferrannini E. Energy Balance After Sodium-Glucose Cotransporter 2 Inhibition. *Diabetes Care*. 2015;38(9):1730-1735. doi:10.2337/dc15-0355

62 Apgar BS, Greenberg G. Using progestins in clinical practice. *Am Fam Physician*. 2000;62(8):1839-1846, 1849-1850.

63 Silva Dos Santos P de N, Madden T, Omvig K, Peipert JF. Changes in body composition in women using long-acting reversible contraception. *Contraception*. 2017;95(4):382-389. 10.1016/j.contraception.2016.12.006

64 Lopez LM, Ramesh S, Chen M, et al. Progestin-only contraceptives: Effects on weight. *Cochrane Database Syst Rev.* 2016;(8):CD008815. 10.1002/14651858.CD008815.pub4

65 Kim CS. Zonisamide effective for weight loss in women. *J Fam Pract.* 2003;52(8):600-601.

66 Pickrell WO, Lacey AS, Thomas RH, Smith PEM, Rees MI. Weight change associated with antiepileptic drugs. *J Neurol Neurosurg Psychiatry.* 2013;84(7):796-799. 10.1136/jnnp-2012-303688

67 Cercato C, Roizenblatt VA, Leanca CC, et al. A randomized double-blind placebo-controlled study of the long-term efficacy and safety of diethylpropion in the treatment of obese subjects. *Int J Obes (Lond).* 2009;33(8):857-865. 10.1038/ijo.2009.124

68 Rodriguez JE, Campbell KM. Past, Present, and Future of Pharmacologic Therapy in Obesity. *Prim Care.* 2016;43(1):61-67, viii. 10.1016/j.pop.2015.08.011

69 Bays HE, Gonzalez-Campoy JM. Adiposopathy. In: *New-Opathies.* WORLD SCIENTIFIC; 2012:105-168. 10.1142/9789814355698_0004

70 Outlaw J, Wilborn C, Smith A, et al. Effects of ingestion of a commercially available thermogenic dietary supplement on resting energy expenditure, mood state and cardiovascular measures. *J Int Soc Sports Nutr.* 2013;10(1):25. 10.1186/1550-2783-10-25

71 Edwards J. How Hydroxycut Stays in Business Despite Deaths, Recalls and a Class-Action Suit. *CBS News.* https://www.cbsnews.com/news/how-hydroxycut-stays-in-business-despite-deaths-recalls-and-a-class-action-suit/. Published June 3, 2011. Accessed June 6, 2019.

72 Saper RB, Eisenberg DM, Phillips RS. Common dietary supplements for weight loss. *Am Fam Physician.* 2004;70(9):1731-1738.

73 Egras AM, Hamilton WR, Lenz TL, Monaghan MS. An evidence-based review of fat modifying supplemental weight loss products. *J Obes.* 2011;2011:297315. doi:10.1155/2011/297315

74 Baltaci D, Deler MH, Turker Y, Ermis F, Iliev D, Velioglu U. Evaluation of serum Vitamin B12 level and related nutritional status among apparently healthy obese female individuals. *Niger J Clin Pract.* 2017;20(1):99-105. 10.4103/1119-

3077.181401

75 Schroeder R, Harrison TD, McGraw SL. Treatment of Adult
Obesity with Bariatric Surgery. *Am Fam Physician*.
2016;93(1):31-37.

76 Dawes AJ, Maggard-Gibbons M, Maher AR, et al. Mental
Health Conditions Among Patients Seeking and Undergoing
Bariatric Surgery: A Meta-analysisMental Health Conditions
Among Bariatric Surgery PatientsMental Health Conditions
Among Bariatric Surgery Patients. *JAMA*. 2016;315(2):150-
163. 10.1001/jama.2015.18118

77 Arterburn D, Wellman R, Emiliano A, et al. Comparative
Effectiveness and Safety of Bariatric Procedures for Weight
Loss: A PCORnet Cohort Study. *Ann Intern Med*.
2018;169(11):741-750. doi:10.7326/M17-2786

78 Kreykes A, Choxi H, Rothberg A. Post-bariatric surgery
patients: Your role in their long-term care. *J Fam Pract*.
2017;66(6):356-363.

Made in the USA
Monee, IL
29 May 2020